A Comprehensive Review of Compartment Syndrome

Edited by Saqeb Beig Mirza and Khaled Elawady

Published in London, United Kingdom

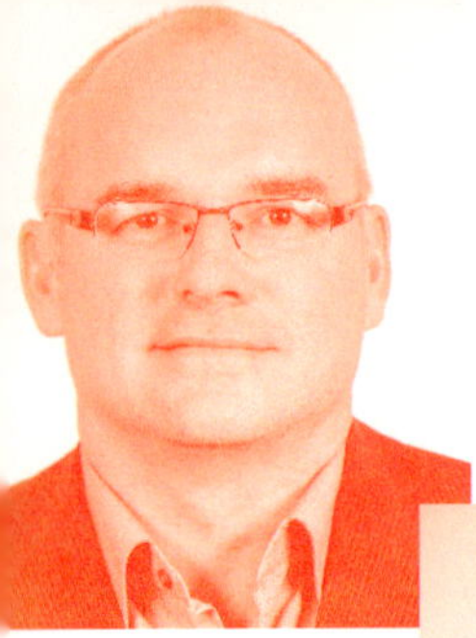
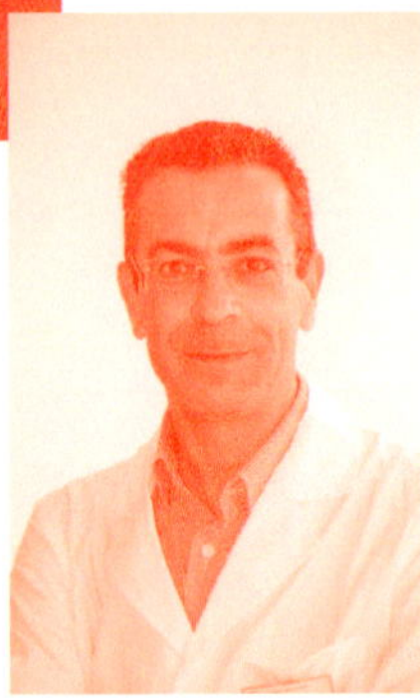
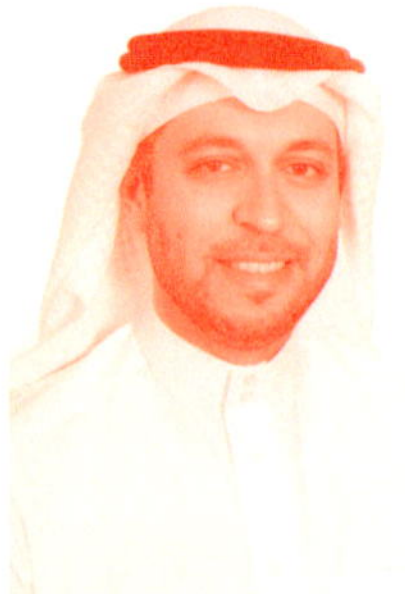
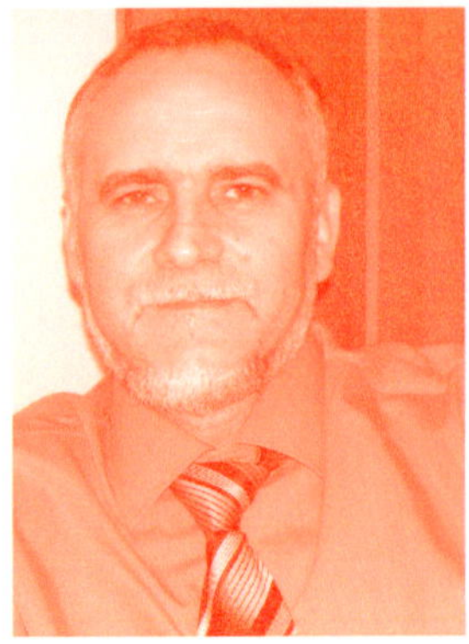
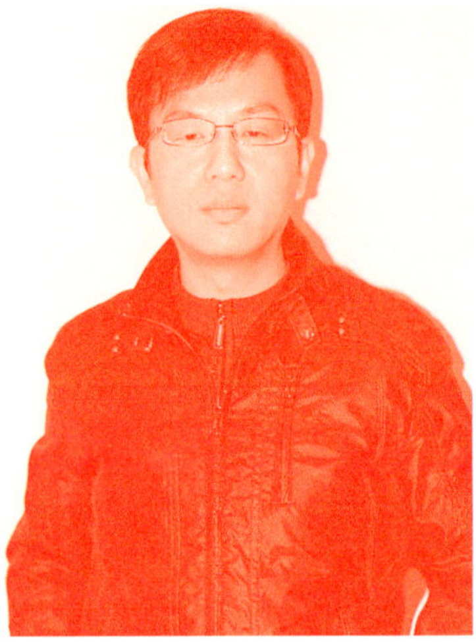
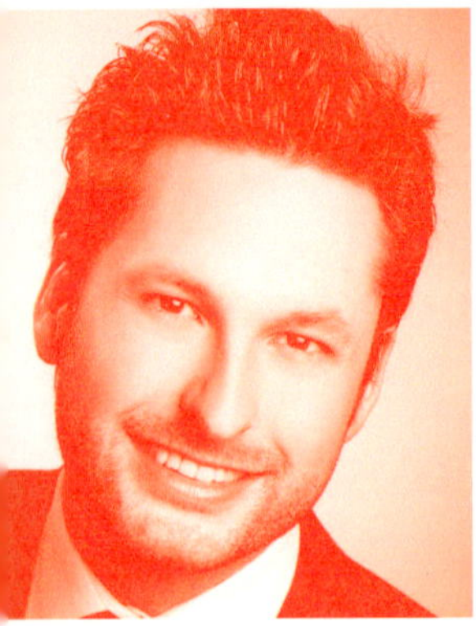
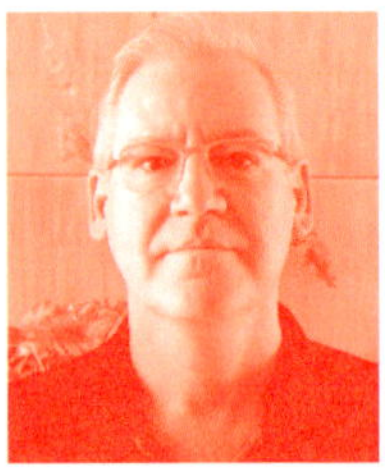

IntechOpen

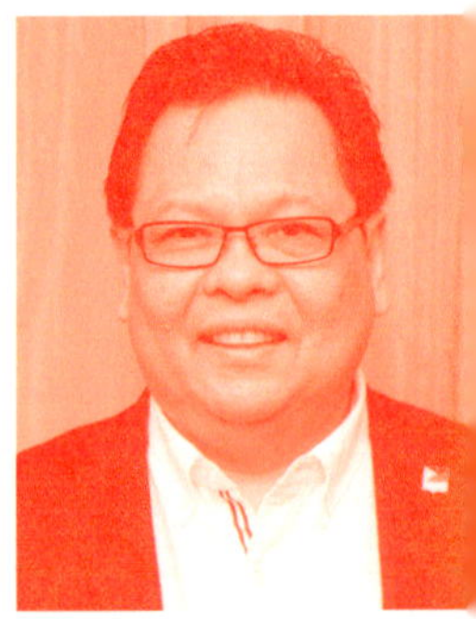
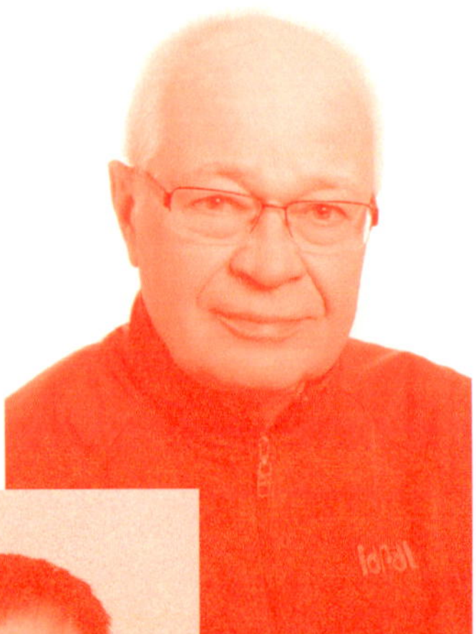
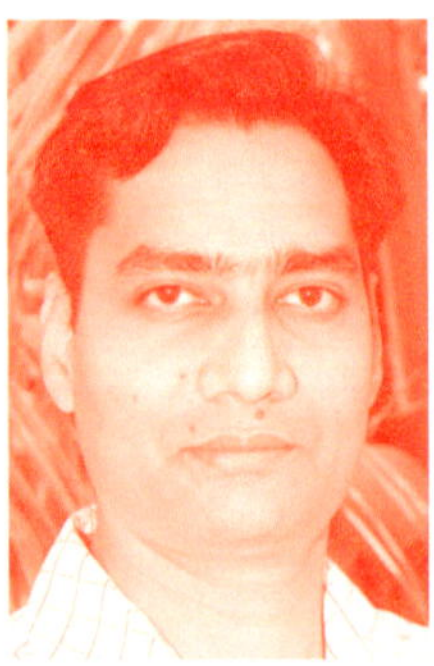
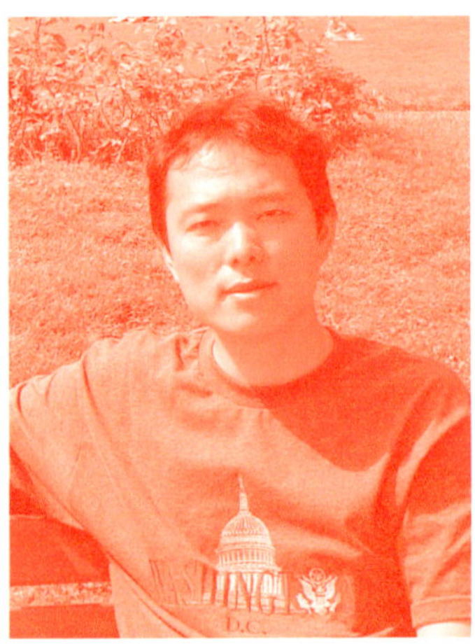
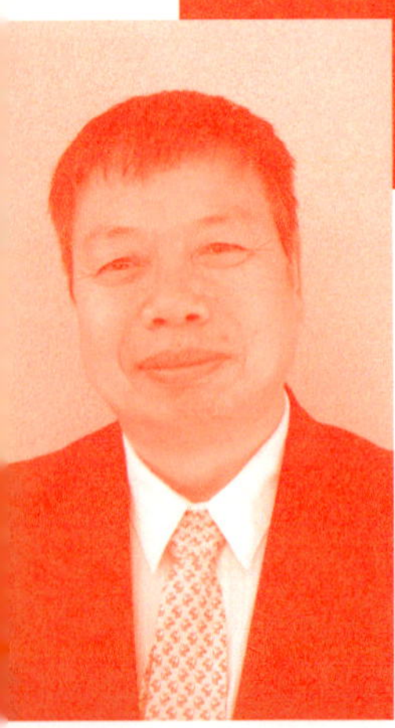
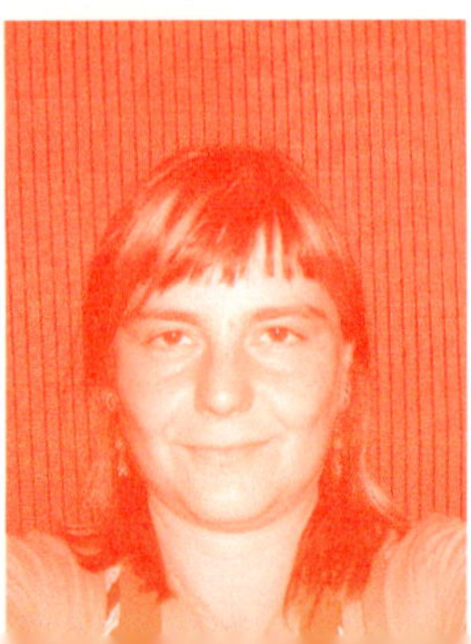

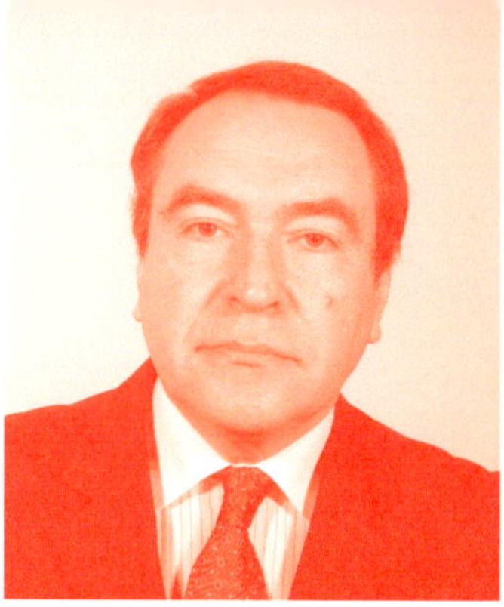

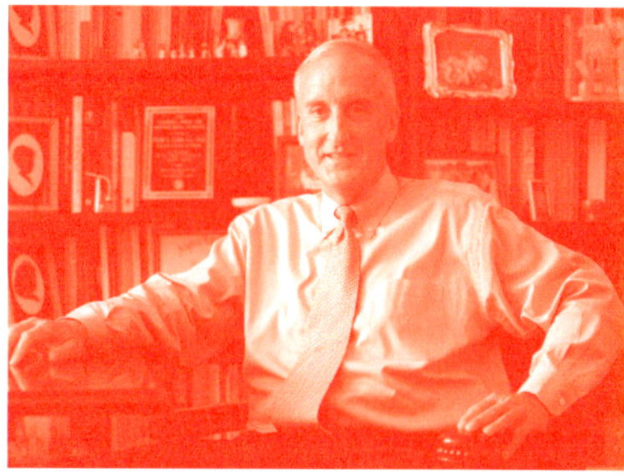

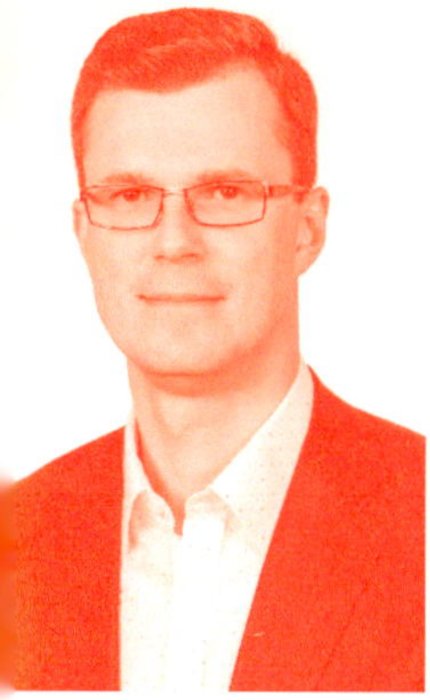

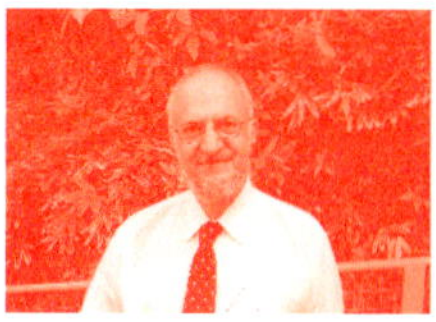

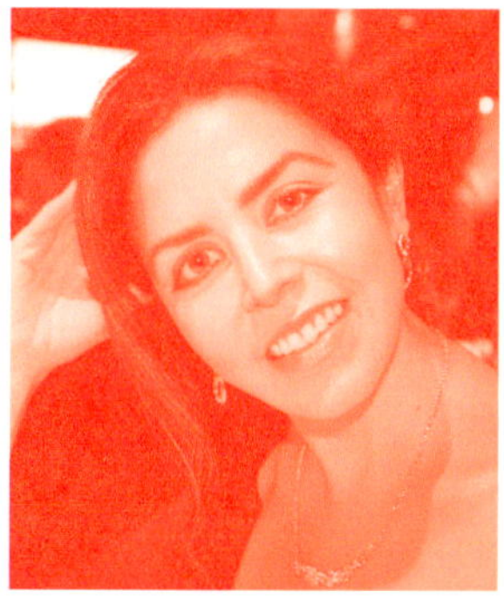

Supporting open minds since 2005

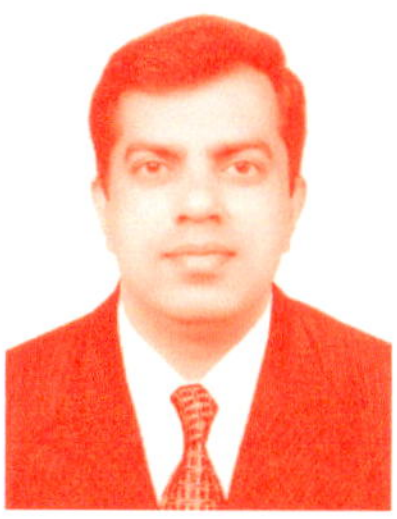

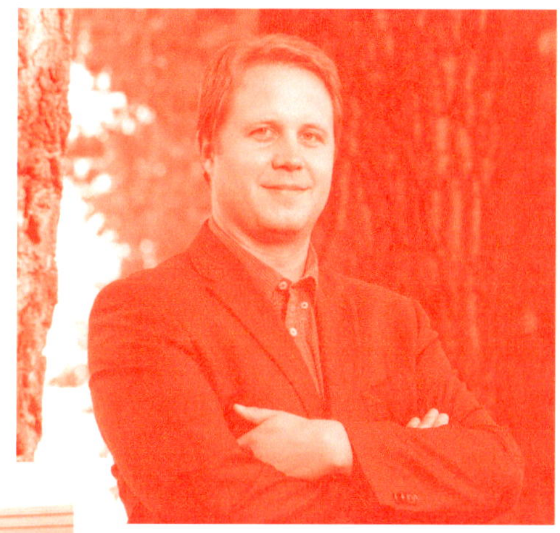

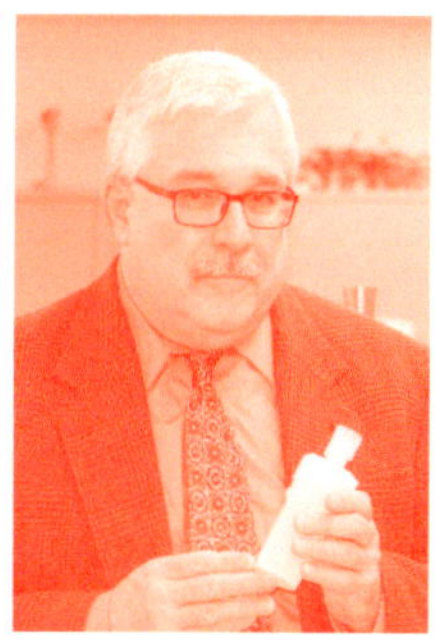

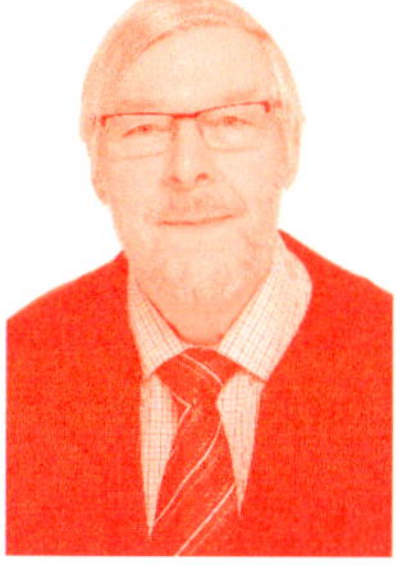

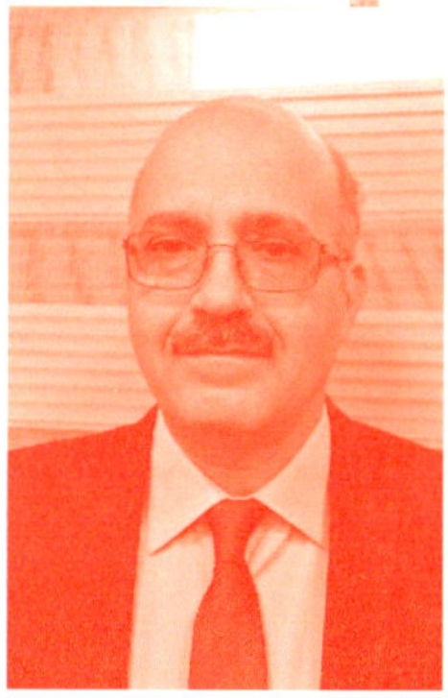

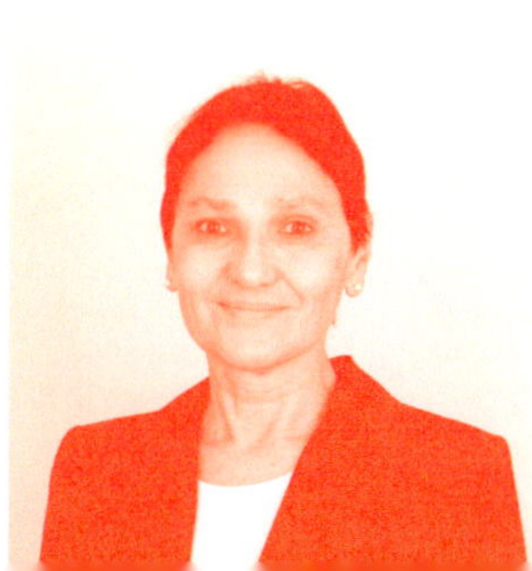

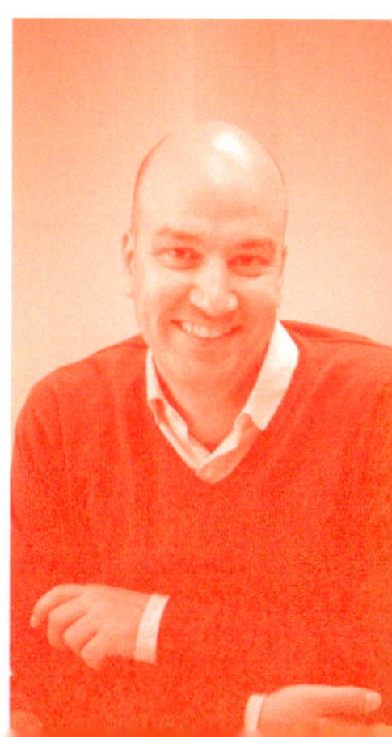

A Comprehensive Review of Compartment Syndrome
http://dx.doi.org/10.5772/intechopen.87609
Edited by Saqeb Beig Mirza and Khaled Elawady

Contributors
Khaled Elawady, Saqeb Beig Mirza, Ioannis M. M. Stavrakakis, George E. Magarakis, Theodoros H. Tosounidis, Salim Surani, Kejal Gandhi, Pahnwat Tonya Taweesedt, Munish Sharma, Dweep Barbhaya, Kuo-Ching Yuan, Hung-Chang Huang, Chih-Yuan Fu, Abdulaziz Shaher, Richard Martin Sellei, Philipp Kobbe, Frank Hildebrand, Ines Laso-Garcia, Fernando Arias-Fúnez, Gemma Duque-Ruiz, David Díaz-Pérez, Alberto Artiles-Medina, Francisco Javier Burgos-Revilla

First published in London, United Kingdom, 2021 by IntechOpen
IntechOpen is the global imprint of INTECHOPEN LIMITED, registered in England and Wales, registration number: 11086078, 5 Princes Gate Court, London, SW7 2QJ, United Kingdom
Printed in Croatia

British Library Cataloguing-in-Publication Data
A catalogue record for this book is available from the British Library

Additional hard and PDF copies can be obtained from orders@intechopen.com

A Comprehensive Review of Compartment Syndrome
Edited by Saqeb Beig Mirza and Khaled Elawady
p. cm.
Print ISBN 978-1-83969-169-0
Online ISBN 978-1-83969-170-6
eBook (PDF) ISBN 978-1-83969-171-3

For EU product safety concerns:
IN TECH d.o.o., Prolaz Marije Krucifikse Kozulić 3, 51000 Rijeka, Croatia, info@intechopen.com or visit our website at intechopen.com.

Meet the editor

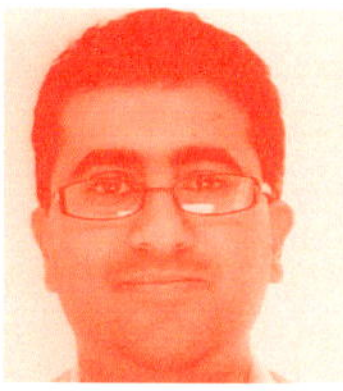

Saqeb Mirza is trauma and orthopedic surgeon currently working at the University Hospital of Wales. His specialist interests are major trauma, foot and ankle, and limb reconstruction. He takes an active interest in research and has authored a number of papers and book chapters in trauma and orthopedic surgery. He also holds an MSc from University College London with a dissertation on the effects of tensile forces on mesenchymal stem cells. He enjoys teaching and training and holds a postgraduate certificate in medical education and a fellowship from the Higher Education Academy, UK. He is an ATLS instructor and holds the FRCS (Tr & Orth), FEBOT and Dip SICOT qualifications.

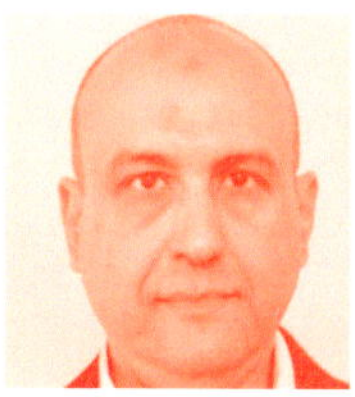

Khaled Elawady is trauma and orthopedic surgeon currently working at the University Hospital of Oxford. His specialist interests are major trauma, pediatric orthopedics and limb reconstruction. He takes an active interest in research and has authored a number of papers and book chapters in trauma and orthopedic surgery. He also holds a Ph.D. and MSc from the University of Cairo. His Ph.D. dissertation was on the congenital absence of leg bones. He enjoys teaching and training and holds a Fellowship of the Royal Colleges of Surgeons (FRCS) in trauma and orthopedics as well as a Membership of the Royal College of Surgeons (MRCS) England.

Contents

Preface

Compartment syndrome is a condition that can be both limb-threatening as well as life-threatening. It often develops in limbs that have been subjected to major trauma, including open injuries. It can develop in any closed osteofascial compartment and its consequences can be devastating to the individual affected.

This book provides a brief synopsis of this very important condition. The first chapter provides an overview of the musculoskeletal compartment syndrome. A section on the musculoskeletal system describes the etiology and pathogenesis of compartment syndrome in detail and looks at the vicious downward spiral that occurs if the condition goes unrecognized, leading to irreversible muscle damage and necrosis. In addition, it looks at the various anatomical sites in the musculoskeletal system in which this condition occurs, acknowledging the need for timely diagnosis. The section also illustrates the various anatomical approaches for decompression of compartments at each site, including the hand and foot.

Compartment syndrome can affect sites other than limbs, with equally devastating complications. The third section discusses these sites, including the thorax and abdomen. It describes the etiologies of the syndrome in these sites, which are many and varied, and provides suggestions for the diagnosis and management of abdominal compartment syndrome.

The fourth section covers the diagnosis of compartment syndrome, which can be challenging. If compartment syndrome is suspected, prompt decompression is generally advocated to save the structures involved from irreversible damage and consequences that may have a significantly negative impact on the patient's life. There are, however, certain situations where compartment pressure monitoring may be useful, for example, in unconscious or ventilated patients. This section describes various methods of compartment pressure monitoring along with their advantages and drawbacks. It also discusses newer methods of diagnosis. However, the current gold standard is still timely clinical examination, a high index of suspicion, and prompt surgical decompression.

The fifth section describes the occurrence of compartment syndrome in special situations. Some of these situations include compartment syndrome in medical patients, those related to patient positioning, and bleeding into compartments in bleeding disorders.

Compartment syndrome remains a condition that can have significant negative consequences for patients if not diagnosed on time. A high index of suspicion is necessary for its diagnosis and time-critical intervention may prevent significant morbidity associated with this condition.

We would like to thank all the authors that contributed to the book as well as IntechOpen Author Service Manager Maja Bozicevic.

Saqeb Beig Mirza
Consultant Trauma and Orthopedic Surgeon,
University Hospital of Wales,
United Kingdom

Khaled Elawady
Fellow,
Trauma and Orthopaedic Surgery,
Oxford University Hospitals,
United Kingdom

Section 1

Introduction

Chapter 1

Review of Compartment Syndrome

Khaled Elawady and Saqeb Beig Mirza

Abstract

Compartment syndrome is a painful condition, caused by increased pressure in a closed muscular compartment. A compartment is a group of muscles enclosed in fascia and septa of connective tissue, which separates different muscle groups. The chambers created receive their blood supply through the arteries. As the pressure builds in the closed space, the blood supply to muscles enclosed decreases. Normal compartment pressure allows blood to flow in and then venous outflow to exit the compartment. However, with increased pressure in the compartment, the arterial flow is impaired. Subsequently, venous outflow stops, adding to the volume of the closed chamber, and hence, pressure builds to the point when the arterial flow stops as well. This chapter provides a general overview of the compartment syndrome in orthopaedic surgical practice. It includes definitions, causes, microscopic anatomy and pathophysiology, as well as the management of this condition.

Keywords: compartment, syndrome, osteofascial, contracture, fasciotomy, plastics, leg compartments

1. Introduction

Compartment syndrome is an acute surgical emergency; it can be limb threatening and potentially life threatening. It results from decreased tissue perfusion secondary to increased pressure within an osteofascial compartment, the consequences of which may result in tissue necrosis. Incidence is more in young men, commonly under 35 years old, and the mean age is different between males (30 years old) and

Males—average age 32 years	91%
Females—average age 44 years	9%
Tibial diaphyseal fracture	36.0%
Soft-tissue injury	23.2%
Distal radial fracture	9.8%
Crush syndrome	7.9%
Diaphyseal fracture of the radius/ulna	7.9%
Femoral fracture	3.0%
Tibial plateau fracture	3.0%

Table 1.
Compartment syndrome risk factors, adapted from [1].

females (44 years old). Sixty-four per cent are associated with fractures, with the annual incidence being 1–7.3 per 100,000 [1].

Acute compartment syndrome affects patients involved in trauma and those patients with associated neurologic and other injuries that can mask the diagnosis. A high degree of suspicion, as well as understanding the natural history and limited value of signs and symptoms, will increase the awareness of the possible diagnosis. The following risk factors can aid in making the diagnosis (**Table 1**) [2].

2. Pathophysiology

Acute compartment syndrome is caused by an increase in the contents of an enclosed space (e.g. bleeding) or a decrease in the volume of a space (e.g. tight cast), or a combination of the two factors. Intercompartmental pressure (ICP) is a function of and an interaction between interstitial pressure and perfusion pressure at the level of the capillary bed. When the interstitial pressure exceeds the perfusion pressure at capillary bed level, there is increased pressure at the venous end of the capillary bed. The resulting increased hydrostatic pressure and further increased intracompartmental pressure eventually limit arteriolar inflow within the system [3]. As a result, the perfusion pressure reduces and ultimately, the perfusion of the compartment stops, leading to anoxia and death of compartment contents (**Figure 1**).

At a cellular level, diminishing ATP levels correlate closely with worsening muscle necrosis, leading to complete muscle necrosis. In a canine study, after 6 h of ischaemia, only 20% of pre-ischaemic ATP remained, which led to complete muscle necrosis [4].

Histologically, there is central muscle necrosis with a surrounding zone of partial ischaemia and peripheral tissue oedema, often within areas of incomplete injury [1]. Adenosine triphosphate (ATP) breakdown occurs as a result of ischaemic injury to the muscle and the severity of this damage is directly related to the level of energy depletion [5].

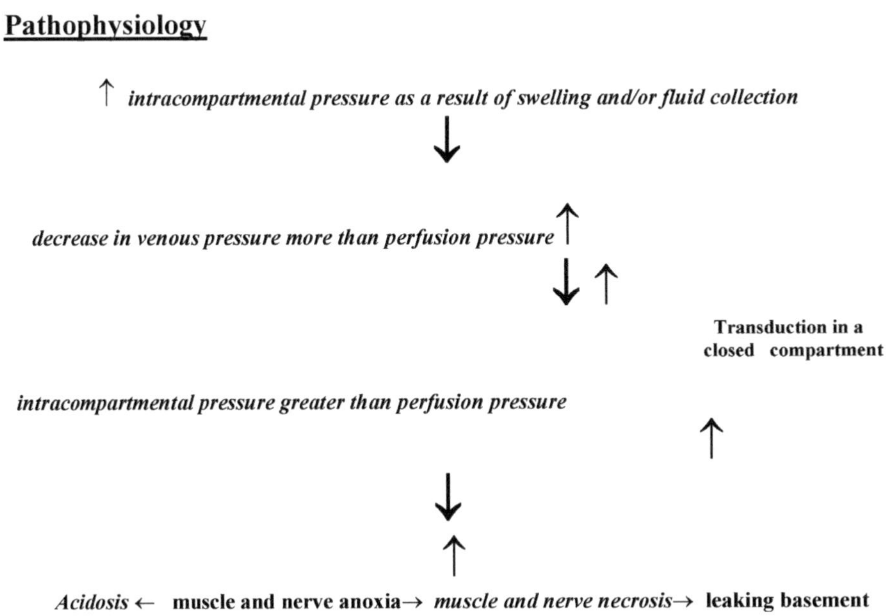

Figure 1.
Illustration of pathophysiologic sequence for the development of acute compartment syndrome.

Skeletal muscles are affected by ischaemia more than other body tissues. With regard to susceptibility to muscle ischaemia, red muscle fibres, for example those located in the anterior compartment of the leg, are more vulnerable to the effects of ischaemia due to their predominant reliance on aerobic metabolic energy in contrast to white muscle fibres, for example the gastrosoleus complex that relies on anaerobically derived energy [6, 7]. Injury (the amount of muscle necrosis) is determined by duration of ischaemia, fibre type, the available residual blood flow and temperature at which ischaemia takes place. Increased collateral blood flow and decreased ischaemic temperature lead to less muscle necrosis [8]. Longer time to diagnose and definitive treatment result in progressive skeletal muscle death and the degree of skeletal muscle injury correlate directly with the severity and duration of ischaemia.

3. Classification

The two main types of compartment syndrome exist, acute and chronic (exertional) compartment syndrome.

Acute compartment syndrome occurs following a fracture, crush injuries, severe muscle bruises, tight casts or bandages, bleeding into compartments in patients with coagulation disorders and heavy drinking or drug abuse.

Chronic exertional compartment syndrome follows repetitive exercise motion and occurs most frequently in people under 40. However, it can develop at any age.

Risk increases with exercises such as swimming, tennis or running, and intense or frequent workouts can also increase the risk. The link between exercise and its association with chronic (exertional) compartment syndrome is not fully understood [9].

4. Diagnosis

There are a few situations that put patients at significant risk of developing compartment syndrome and warrant routine observations for compartment syndrome. These include major limb injuries including open or segmental long-bone injuries caused by high-energy mechanisms, operative management of major limb injuries and prolonged surgical procedures that may compromise or affect limb perfusion adversely. In these cases, it should be routine procedure to monitor the limb closely for any signs of evolving compartment syndrome.

The BOAST guidelines recommend meticulous documentation of the clinical findings in suspected compartment syndrome. In addition, it is important to record the mechanism of injury and the time it occurred as well as the initial time of evaluation and ongoing clinical reviews. Pain levels and analgesic requirements should be recorded and whether or not any regional anaesthetics had been used thus far [10].

The most important and diagnostically significant signs include pain on passive stretch of the muscles in the individual compartments affected and pain out of proportion to the injury, and these should be acted upon in a timely manner [1, 2].

Documentation of neural function and vascular perfusion including capillary refill time and pulses need to be recorded and documented even though they have little role in the early and timely diagnosis of an evolving acute compartment syndrome [10].

Classic features including pain, pallor, pulselessness, paraesthesia, poikilothermia and paralysis are more considered late signs of a limb that has been vascularly compromised and do not really play a part in early diagnosis of ACS [11]. Undiagnosed acute compartment syndrome will cause progressive muscle damage.

Therefore, it may be beneficial for one experienced assessor to serially examine the patient, so the evolution of the condition is noted rather than at one point in time and at the same time avoid interobserver error [11, 12].

The presence of all five features may indicate a late diagnosis and irreversible damage because some features such as paralysis occur very late in the pathogenesis of acute compartment syndrome. Frequent serial clinical assessment must be interpreted taking into consideration the patient's individual risk [11].

When compartment pressure measurements are indicated, for example in unconscious patients, the diastolic blood pressure is recorded. If the difference between diastolic blood pressure and compartment pressure is less than 30 mmHg, this suggests an increased risk of compartment syndrome and a decision should be made either to proceed to surgical decompression or to continue monitoring. This decision-making process should involve a senior clinician [10].

Bayes' theorem has been used to calculate the predictive values of some of the cardinal features of acute compartment syndrome. These included pain, paraesthesia, paresis and pain on passive movement of the muscles involved. The high specificity and negative predictive values for these factors suggested that their absence correlated with a less likelihood of the presence of an acute compartment syndrome, but they had a low-positive predictive value indicating that presence of these symptoms on their own had a low correlation with acute compartment syndrome [13].

5. Management

The initial management should involve splitting the plaster dressing to skin level. Studies have shown that removing dressings overlying the compartment suspected of raised ICP, splitting the cast reduced ICP by a mean of 65% [14]. Moreover, a 10–20% further reduction occurred after the padding cut to skin level. However, even after the removal of tight casts, continued monitoring for clinical features of ACS should occur and it is recommended that the limb should not be elevated excessively but rather be maintained at heart level to perfuse the compartment [14].

If acute compartment syndrome clinical features do not regress following this, a fasciotomy indicated and should be carried out as an emergency procedure [15]. In some special situations, fasciotomy may not be indicated, for example in patients who already have muscle death due to muscle crush syndrome suffered in situations such as natural disasters. In these cases, conservative management may be more appropriate in these patients. The decision to proceed with fasciotomy was based on a comprehensive clinical assessment [16].

In certain circumstances, some authors consider primary amputation a better option than decompressive fasciotomy, especially if there has been a duration of greater than 8 h following the onset of symptoms of acute compartment syndrome with absent muscle function [17].

Compartment pressure measurement can be used as an adjunct to clinical examination, especially if the clinical symptoms cannot be elicited, for example in unconscious or ventilated patients, or if clinical examination is equivocal, or unreliable [17].

Serial compartment pressure measurement, with the initial measure used as a reference point, detects a further rise in the compartment pressure [1].

Two standard techniques for compartment pressure measurement are the slit catheter and the side-port needle. The slit catheter is a low-volume infusion technique [18]. The catheter may be left within the compartment for repeated or continuous compartment pressure measurements for hours.

Side-port needles can be used to measure multiple compartments, and studies have shown no significant difference statistically when comparing the measurements taken with a slit catheter or the side-port needle [19].

Using an18-gauge needle to measure intracompartmental pressure tends to overestimate the value of the intracompartmental pressure by 20 mmHg when compared with the slit catheter method or the side-port needle and may hence be less accurate. Several commercially available pressure measurement devices are available for determining the intracompartmental pressures.

There is a relationship between compartmental tissue pressure and the distance from the site of the fracture. In one study, the highest pressure recorded was in the deep posterior or anterior compartments, or both, and 89% of compartments had the highest pressure measurement at the fracture site [20].

Once an impending or confirmed compartment syndrome diagnosis has been made, immediate measures necessary must be taken to reduce the chances of progression. These include splitting or taking any casts or occlusive dressings off. Cast padding or circumferential dressings have to be released around their entire circumference, and the limb has to be elevated to the level of the patient's heart to maximise perfusion while minimising swelling. If, in spite of these steps, the clinical signs of compartment syndrome do not resolve, emergent and complete fasciotomy of all compartments with elevated pressures is necessary.

Patients should be counselled about the risks associated with fasciotomy such as wound healing problems, weakness, chronic venous insufficiency, non-union of the associated fractures and subsequent plastic surgical intervention, for example skin grafting.

There are several techniques of decompression for different parts of the body.

5.1 Forearm compartment syndrome

There are three compartments: the volar compartment (superficial and deep), dorsal compartment and mobile wad of Henry (lateral) compartments.

Decompression of all involved compartments is mandatory, involves a volar incision 1 cm proximal and 2 cm lateral to the medial epicondyle and obliquely crosses the antecubital fossa and over the volar aspect of the mobile wad, and then curves medially, reaching the midline at the junction of the middle and distal third of the forearm and continued just medial to the palmaris longus tendon to avoid the palmar cutaneous branch of the median nerve incision, crossing the wrist crease at an angle and extending into the mid-palm for a carpal tunnel release if necessary (**Figure 2**).

The lacertus fibrosus and fascia overlying the flexor carpi ulnaris must be opened and flexor carpi ulnaris is retracted ulnarly, and the flexor digitorum superficialis is retracted radially to permit opening of the fascia of the deep volar compartment, avoiding the ulnar nerve and artery carefully during dissection.

Dorsal compartment release is through a longitudinal incision 2 cm distal to the lateral epicondyle towards the midline of the wrist, dissecting between the interval of extensor digitorum communis and extensor carpi radialis brevis. The muscles of the forearm should be palpated and if soft, no further procedure should be performed. If residual muscle tension is felt, then an epimysiotomy is performed.

5.2 Hand compartment syndrome

In the hand, 10 compartments may be affected by rising compartment pressures. They are hypothenar, thenar, adductor pollicis, dorsal interosseous (four) and volar interosseous (three).

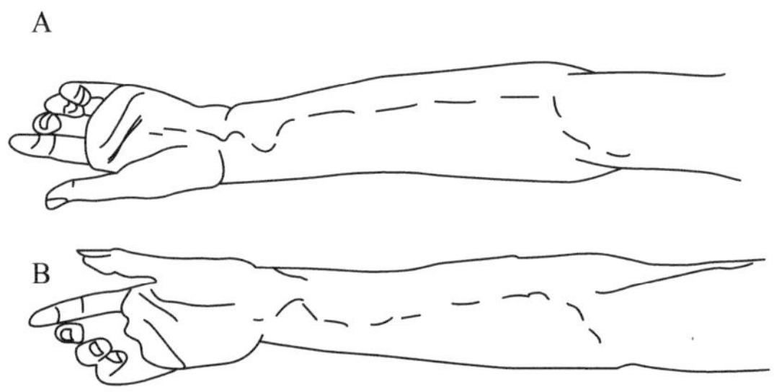

Figure 2.
Illustration of the incisions used to decompress the volar forearm.

Release of the volar and dorsal interosseous compartments and the adductor compartment to the thumb is done with two longitudinal incisions dorsally over the second and fourth metacarpals (**Figure 3**).

Incising the fascia over the dorsal interosseous muscles and blunt dissection is performed along the ulnar side of the second metacarpal to decompress the first volar interosseous through the more radial incision, and the radial aspect of the fourth and fifth metacarpals is dissected through an ulnar incision to release the second and third volar interosseous compartments. For releasing the thenar and hypothenar compartments, longitudinal incisions are made at the junctions of the glabrous and non-glabrous skin over the radial side of the first metacarpal and the ulnar side of the fifth metacarpal.

Ideally, hand fasciotomies should be done by a hand surgeon unless there is an immediate need with no access to a hand surgeon [21].

Various locations in the lower extremity can develop compartment syndromes, for example the gluteal musculature, the muscles of the thigh and lower leg, and foot.

Early recognition and decompression are the key to avoid long-term complications and even amputation of the limb.

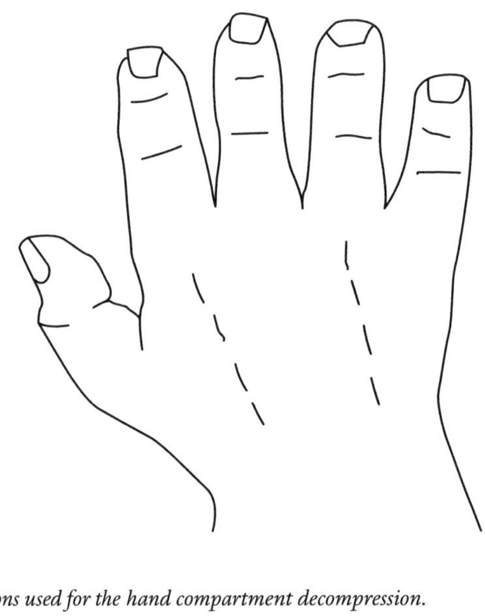

Figure 3.
Drawing of the two incisions used for the hand compartment decompression.

5.3 Gluteal musculature

Posterior incision decompresses the gluteus maximus and the abductor musculature used sufficiently to decompress the gluteal region.

5.4 Thigh compartment syndrome

A long single lateral incision can sufficiently decompress the anterior and posterior compartments of the thigh. A medial adductor incision may be required if ongoing symptoms of increased compartment pressure are evident despite adequate decompression through the long lateral incision.

5.5 Leg compartment syndrome

The length of the skin incision influences fascial decompression in the leg associated with an acute compartment syndrome, to normalise the compartment pressures and restore perfusion to the tissues. Some authors favour limited incisions, claiming low morbidity, while others recommend long incisions, emphasising that these are required to decompress the affected compartment adequately [17].

In a trauma situation, long incisions are recommended for adequate decompression. Hyperaemia post-decompression is avoided by using long incisions to prevent the skin from creating a tight compartment envelope [22].

Leg decompression can be done *via* a one-incision or a two-incision approach.

The one-incision technique, although described, is difficult and not widely used. It involves a long single lateral incision over the anterolateral leg made 5 cm of distal to the head of the fibula and proximal to the lateral malleolus [22]. This is followed by identifying the septum between the anterior and lateral compartments and avoiding the injury to the superficial peroneal nerve distally, the anterior and lateral compartments on either side of the septum are decompressed [23].

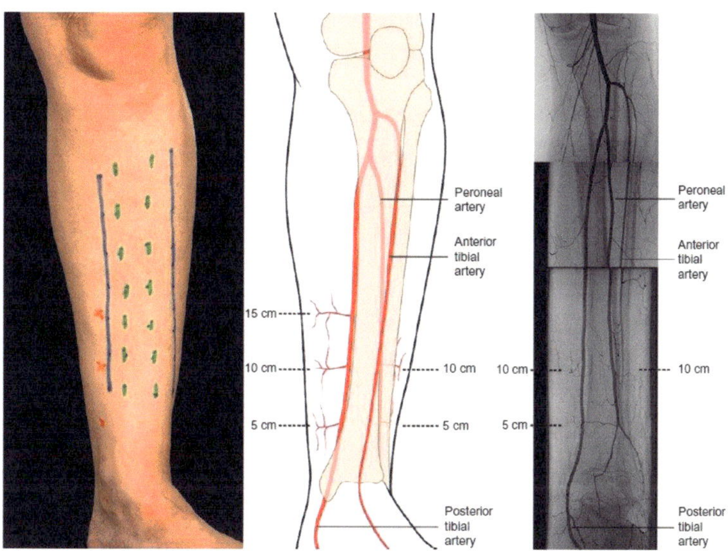

Figure 4.
Two-incision fasciotomies; the medial incision alone is usually sufficient for debridement and preserves the perforators arising from the posterior tibial vessels, which form the basis of local fasciocutaneous flaps.

Then, the lateral compartment musculature is lifted from the intramuscular septum and incising the intramuscular septum to access the lateral portion of the superficial posterior compartment, and through this incision, the deep posterior compartment can be decompressed by mobilising the superficial compartment posteriorly [17].

The more widely used and accepted approach is a two-incision technique (**Figure 4**), and this is the approach recommended in the UK BOAST/BAPRAS guidelines.

The location of the medial skin incision is crucial as muscles in the superficial posterior compartment are proximal and the incision needs to reach the proximal part of the deep posterior compartment to decompress these muscles adequately.

The leg deep posterior musculature is on the other hand in the distal half of the limb and decompressing them involves detaching the soleus origin from the medial aspect of the tibial shaft. Extra care is taken at this point as posterior tibial neurovascular bundle lies just deep to the investing fascia. A careful assessment of muscle viability is needed, and all non-viable muscles should be excised.

It should be noted that the lateral incision, if inadvertently placed over the fibula (too lateral), can expose the periosteum, and if placed too far distally, the incision can expose the peroneal tendons, exposing bone and/or tendons increase incidence of infection and delayed healing, and may end in amputation [20].

5.6 Foot compartment syndrome

Foot compartment syndrome is a controversial subject, as some foot and ankle specialists advocate not interfering surgically due to the associated morbidity with surgery.

In the foot, there are nine main compartments: medial, lateral, interosseous (four) and central (three), and dual dorsal incisions are recommended for decompression of the foot compartments (**Figure 5**).

A dorsal medial incision is made medial to second metatarsal, and this releases the first and second interosseous, medial and deep central compartment.

The dorsal lateral incision is made lateral to the fourth metatarsal and releases the third and fourth interosseous, lateral, superficial and middle central compartments.

To do this, the dorsal fascia of each interosseous compartment is opened longitudinally, muscles stripped from the medial fascia of the first interosseous compartment, split adductor compartment and a medial incision may be added

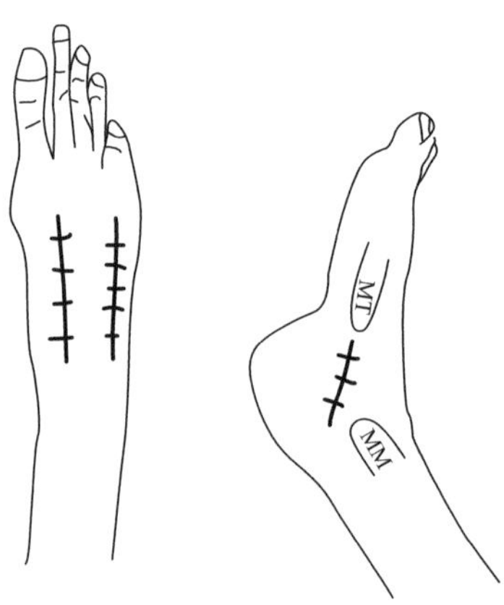

Figure 5.
Drawing depicts the two dorsal and medial incisions used to decompress the foot compartments.

for decompression of calcaneal compartment with the release of the fascia of the intrinsic foot muscles at their metatarsal attachments [24, 25].

6. Conclusion

Acute compartment syndrome is an acute limb-threatening condition. Its diagnosis is mainly clinical and involves certain cardinal features. A high index of suspicion is needed to make the diagnosis. The condition is time critical and timely surgical intervention is the key to success.

Abbreviations

ICP	intracompartmental pressure
ACS	acute compartment syndrome

Author details

Khaled Elawady[1]* and Saqeb Beig Mirza[2]

1 Oxford University Hospital, UK

2 University Hospital of Wales, UK

*Address all correspondence to: kaledawady@gmail.com

References

[1] McQueen MM, Gaston P, Court-Brown CM. A molecular interaction database. Acute compartment syndrome. Who is at risk? The Journal of Bone and Joint Surgery. British Volume. 2000;**82**(2):200-203

[2] McQueen MM, Christie J, Court-Brown CM. Compartment pressures after intramedullary nailing of the tibia. The Journal of Bone and Joint Surgery. British Volume. 1990;**72**: 395-397

[3] Tiwari A, Hag AI, Myint F, et al. Acute compartment syndromes. Journal of British Surgery. 2002;**89**:397-412. DOI: 10.1046/j.0007-1323.2002.02063. x

[4] Hayes G, Liauw S, Romaschin A, et al. Separation of reperfusion injury from ischemia-induced necrosis. Surgical Forum. 1988;**39**:306-308

[5] Lindsay T, Liauw F, Romaschin S, et al. The effect of ischemia/reperfusion on adenine nucleotide metabolism and xanthine oxidase production in skeletal muscle. Journal of Vascular Surgery. 1990;**12**:8-15

[6] Blaisdell FW. The pathophysiology of skeletal muscle ischemia and the reperfusion syndrome: A review. Cardiovascular Surgery. 2002;**10**:620-630. DOI: 10.1016/S0967-2109(02)00070-4

[7] Jennische E. Ischemia-induced injury in glycogen-depleted skeletal muscle: Selective vulnerability of the FG-fibres. Acta Physiologica Scandinavica. 1985;**125**:727-734. DOI: 10.1111/j.1748-1716.1985.tb07776.x

[8] Petrasek PF, Homer-Vanniasinkam S, Walker PM. Determinants of ischemic injury to skeletal muscle. Journal of Vascular Surgery. 1994;**19**:623-631. DOI: 10.1016/S0741-5214(94)70035-4

[9] Bae DS, Kadiyala RK, Waters PM. Acute compartment syndrome in children: Contemporary diagnosis, treatment, and outcomes. Journal of Pediatric Orthopaedics. 2001;**21**:680-688. DOI: 10.1097/00004694-200109000-00025

[10] BOAST British Orthopaedic Association Standards for Trauma. Review date: December 2016. For correspondence, contact: policy@boa.ac.u

[11] Malik AA, Khan WS, Chaudhry A, et al. Acute compartment syndrome a life and limb-threatening surgical emergency. Journal of Perioperative Practice. 2009;**19**(5):137-142

[12] Shuler FD, Dietz MJ. Physicians' ability to manually detect isolated elevations in leg intracompartmental pressure. The Journal of Bone & Joint Surgery. 2010;**92**(2):361-367

[13] Ulmer T. The clinical diagnosis of compartment syndrome of the lower leg: Are clinical findings predictive of the disorder? Journal of Orthopaedic Trauma. 2002;**16**(8):572-577

[14] Köstler W, Strohm PC, Südkamp NP. Acute compartment syndrome of the limb. Injury. 2004;**35**(12):1221-1227

[15] Murphy JB. Myositis. JAMA: The Journal of the American Medical Association. 1914;**63**:1249

[16] Mubarak SJ, Hargens AR. Acute compartment syndromes. Surgical Clinics of North America. 1983;**63**(3):539-565

[17] Olson SA, Glasgow RR. Acute compartment syndrome in lower extremity musculoskeletal trauma. Journal of the American Academy of Orthopaedic Surgeons. 2005;**13**(7): 436-444

[18] Shakespeare DT, Henderson NJ, Clough G. The slit catheter: A comparison with the wick catheter in the measurement of compartment pressure. Injury. 1982;**13**:404-408

[19] Moed BR, Thorderson PK. Measurement of intracompartmental pressure: A comparison of the slit catheter, side-ported needle, and simple needle. The Journal of Bone and Joint Surgery: American Volume. 1993;**75**: 231-235

[20] Heckman MM, Whitesides TE Jr, Grewe SR, et al. Compartment pressure in association with closed tibial fractures: The relationship between tissue pressure, compartment, and the distance from the site of the fracture. The Journal of Bone and Joint Surgery. American Volume. 1994;**76**:1285-1292

[21] Ouellette EA. Compartment syndromes in obtunded patients. Hand Clinics. 1998;**14**(3):431-450

[22] Cohen MS, Garfin SR, Hargens AR, et al. Acute compartment syndrome: Effect of dermotomy on fascial decompression in the leg. The Journal of Bone and Joint Surgery. British Volume. 1991;**73**:287-290

[23] Purcell D, Terry BA, Sharp BR. Acute compartment syndrome. In: Purcell D, Chinai S, Allen B, Davenport M, editors. Emergency Orthopedics Handbook. Cham: Springer; 2019. DOI: 10.1007/978-3-030-00707-2_3

[24] Sigamoney K, Khincha P, Badge R, et al. Compartment syndrome: Challenges and solutions. Orthopedic Research and Reviews. 2015;7:137-148. DOI: 10.2147/ORR.S50776

[25] Prasarn ML, Ouellette EA. Acute compartment syndrome of the upper extremity. J Am Acad Orthop Surg. 2011 Jan;19(1):49-58. doi: 10.5435/00124635-201101000-00006. Erratum in: J Am Acad Orthop Surg. 2011 May;19(5):50A. PMID: 21205767.

Section 2

Compartment Syndrome in Musculoskeletal Sites

Chapter 2

Hand Compartment Syndrome

Ioannis M. Stavrakakis, George E. Magarakis and Theodoros H. Tosounidis

Abstract

Compartment syndrome is defined by high pressures in a closed myofascial compartment, which affects initially the muscles and later the nerves and vessels. The hand is rarely affected, but if treated suboptimally, it results to a permanent loss of function. Eleven compartments are included in the hand and wrist. Diagnosis of compartment syndrome of the hand remains challenging. Pain out of proportion of injury and excessive swelling should raise suspicion towards a compartment syndrome. Intracompartmental pressure measurement contributes to the diagnosis, but it is not always reliable. Once the diagnosis of acute compartment syndrome has been made, decompression of all compartments is mandatory, in order to achieve a good outcome. Failing to manage this emergent condition properly leads to a significant hand disability. Our chapter includes the following sections: 1. Introduction. A brief description of the hand compartment syndrome is presented. 2. Anatomy. Special considerations regarding hand compartments are presented, 3. Etiology. 4. Diagnosis. Signs and symptoms are reported, as well as guidelines of the technique of intracompartmental pressure measurement. 5. Treatment. Faciotomies' indications and operative technique are described in details. 6. Conclusion. Appropriate figures of the clinical image and surgical decompression are presented as well.

Keywords: hand, compartment syndrome, intracompartmental pressure, surgical decompression, fasciotomy

1. Introduction

Compartment syndrome is defined as an elevated pressure of an anatomical compartment up to a level where the tissue blood perfusion is impeded. Acute compartment syndrome (ACS) of the hand is rare, as compared to other areas of the human body, but the consequences are detrimental if treated suboptimally. Severe functional disability of the hand, due to muscles' contractures, is the inevitable result of a neglected compartment syndrome. Diagnosis of this urgent situation is challenging and it is based mainly on the clinical examination [1–3].

In case there is any doubt towards the diagnosis of ACS or for insensate patients, intracompartmental pressure measurement is used to aid the evaluation [4]. Good knowledge of the special anatomy of the hand is necessary, in order to manage compartment syndrome appropriately. Disproportionate pain, severe swelling and a relevant mechanism should raise a strong suspicion of a compartment syndrome [5]. Once the diagnosis of an ACS is made, treatment should be implemented promptly. Intervention varies from simple actions, such as splitting a tight cast, to a surgical decompression [2]. Correct timing of fasciotomies is of paramount importance, in order to achieve a good functional outcome [6].

This chapter aims to present the current concepts regarding hand compartment syndrome. Special features of the hand compartments' anatomy are reported. Pathophysiology is described briefly, as it is analyzed in extension in other parts of this book. Etiology, diagnosis, treatment and complications are mentioned as well, emphasizing towards the proper technique of fasciotomies.

2. Anatomy - pathophysiology

Hand contains basically ten myofascial compartments: the adductor pollicis compartment, four dorsal interossei and three palmar interossei compartments, the thenar and the hypothenar compartment. The thenar compartment includes the Abductor Pollicis Brevis (AbPB), the Flexor Pollicis Brevis (FPB) and the Opponens Pollicis (OP) muscles. They are innervated by the recurrent motor branch of the median nerve, apart from the deep head of the FPB, which is innervated by the deep branch of the ulnar nerve [2]. The hypothenar compartment includes the Opponens Digiti Minimi (ODM), the Abductor Digiti Minimi (AbDM) and Flexor Digiti Minimi (FDM) muscles. They are all innervated by branches of the ulnar nerve (**Figure 1**). Although located basically in the wrist, the carpal tunnel is frequently mentioned as a compartment of the hand. Cleland and Grayson ligaments also compartmentalize digital space. All compartments of the hand along with their muscles and nerves are presented on the **Table 1** [2, 4, 7]. It is highlighted here that the compartments of the hand contain predominantly motor nerves. Intracompartmental sensory nerves of the hand are only the digital nerves and the median nerve inside the carpal tunnel. This characteristic anatomy is reflected to the clinical image of the compartment syndrome of the hand [4, 5, 8].

Several variations of the hand compartments have been described. Difelice et al. [7] found that in 52% of the hands, the thenar space is separated in two discrete compartments. In 76% of the hands the hypothenar demonstrated at least two compartments. The second, third and fourth interossei group demonstrated different dorsal and volar compartment in the 48%, 67% and 38% of the hands respectively. The fasciotomies used for the treatment of hand ACS are designed based on this anatomic

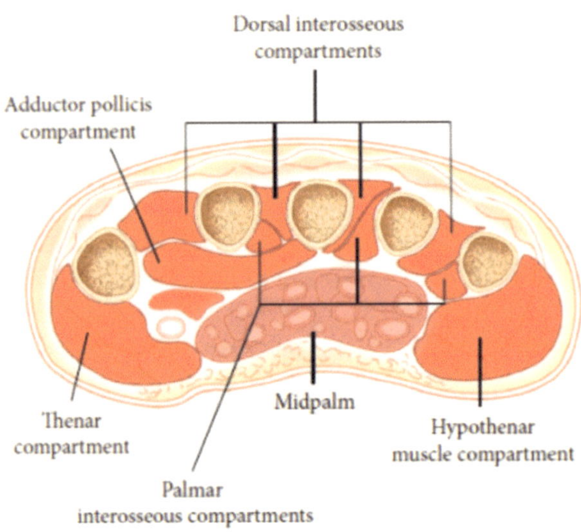

Figure 1.
Hand compartments cross sectional anatomy. (from: Reichman EF. Compartment syndrome of the hand: A little thought about diagnosis. Case rep Emerg med. 2016;2016 [5]).

Compartment	Muscles	Nerves	Incision
Adductor Pollicis	Adductor Pollicis	Sensory: None Motor: Branches of the ulnar nerve	Dorsal over the second metacarpal (radial aspect)
Interossei compartments	4 dorsal interossei, 3 palmar interossei	Sensory: None Motor: Branches of the ulnar nerve	Two Dorsal incsions over the second and fourth metacarpal
Thenar	AbPB, OP, FPB	Sensory: None Motor: Recurrent motor branch of the median nerve, apart from the deep head of the FBP (ulnar nerve)	Radial aspect of the first metacarpal
Hypothenar	AbDM, FDM, ODM	Sensory: None Motor: Ulnar nerve	Ulnar aspect of the fifth metacarpal
Carpal tunnel	None (FPL, 4 FDS, 4 FDP tendons/not muscles)	Sensory: Median nerve Motor: Recurrent motor branch of the median nerve	Midpalmar incision
Digital	None (digital tendons/not muscles)	Sensory: digital nerves Motor: None	Lateral midaxial incision

AbPB: abductor pollicis brevis, OP: opponens pollicis, FPB: flexor pollicis brevis, AbDM: abductor digiti minimi, FDM: flexor digiti minimi, ODM: opponens digiti minimi, FPL: flexor pollicis longus, FDS: flexor digitorum superficialis, FDP: flexor digitorum profoundis.

Table 1.
Compartments of the hand.

model. Whether further subcompartmentalization of the thenar and hypothenar area has any clinical significance is controversial. Gyuton et al. [9] found through a cadaveric study that fascia between dorsal and volar interrossei muscles subsides at pressures as low as 15 mmHg, putting its clinical relevance in question.

The pathophysiology of acute compartment syndrome is based on Matsen's arteriovenous gradient theory. According to this model, interstitial edema increases the local venous pressure (Pv). Local blood flow (LBF) equals to arteriovenous pressure difference (Pa - Pv), divided by vascular resistance (R). Thus, the increase of the local venous pressure decreases local blood flow. Tissue ischemia increases small vessels permeability as well as extravascular osmolality, leading to a further fluid extravasation and subsequent more interstitial edema. Viscious cycle is continued through the former mechanism. Local and systemic inflammatory response is exacerbated by the release of cytokines, as a result of impaired tissue blood supply [4, 10].

Muscle damage due to compartment syndrome occurs prior to nerve impairment and it is reversible for the first 4 hours. The time frame after which muscle necrosis is occurred is still controversial, with a reported range among studies between 8 to 12 hours [2, 4, 11]. Experimental studies of canine model showed permanent tissue necrosis and nerve conduction arrest with interstitial pressures of more than 40 mmHg for at least 8 hours [12].

3. Etiology

Intracompartmental pressure increases by either extrinsic or intrinsic causes or combination of both. Tight dressings or casts represent extrinsic factors, via external pressure application to the compartments of the hand [13].

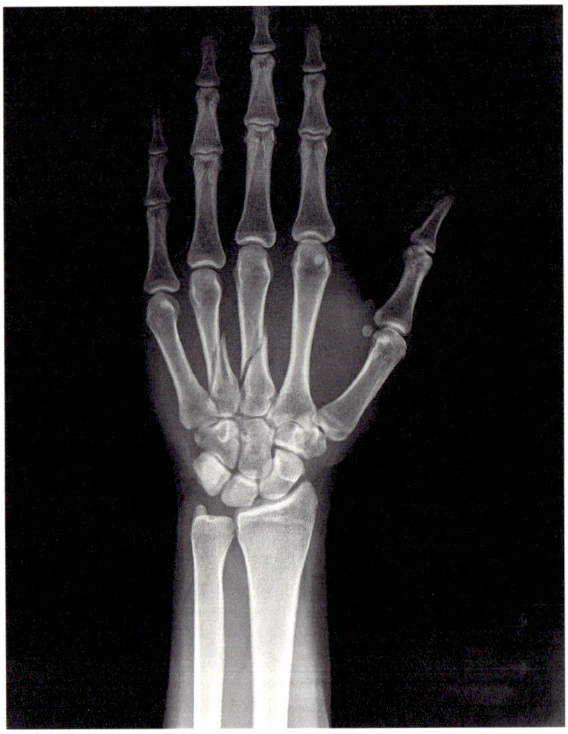

Figure 2.
Hand crush syndrome. Compartment syndrome due to extensive soft tissue injury and concomitant third and fourth metacarpal fractures, after prolonged compression of the hand by a heavy object.

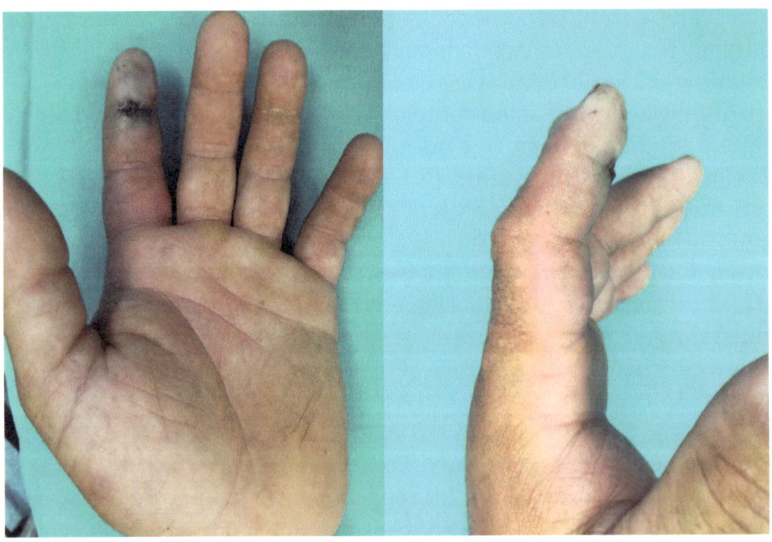

Figure 3.
Index finger compartment syndrome (delayed presentation), due to high pressure injection injury, complicated with septic tenosynovitis.

Intrinsic causes of hand compartment syndrome are:

1. Trauma: fractures, soft tissue injury, crush syndrome (**Figure 2**),

2. Burns,

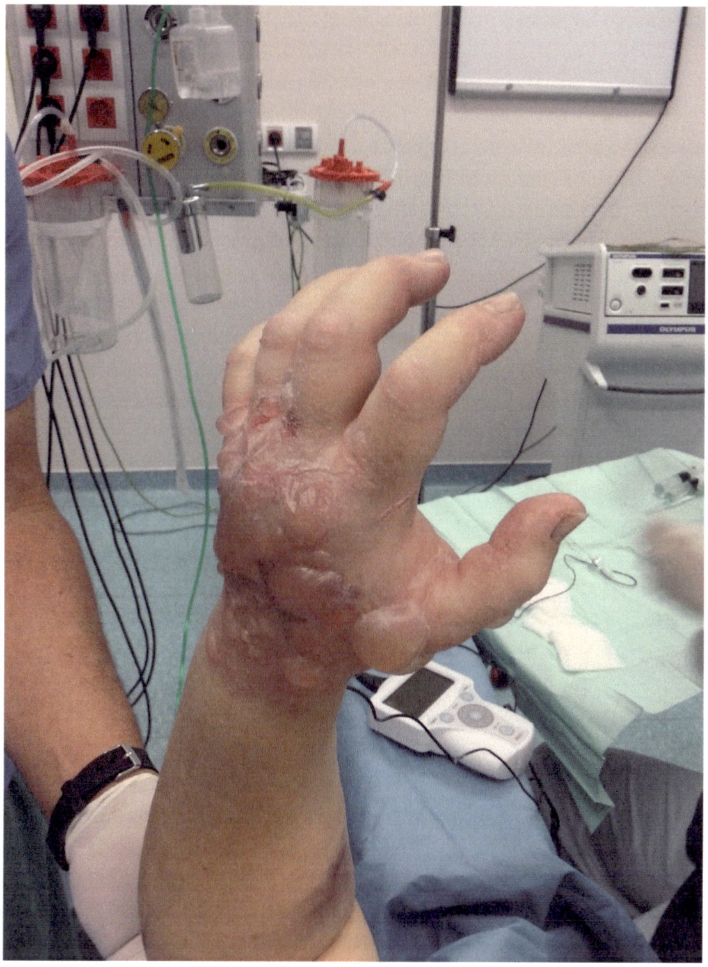

Figure 4.
Hand compartment syndrome due to extravasation contrast material. Hand is sitting in intrinsic minus position. Excessive swelling and skin blisters are noticed (from: Stavrakakis IM et al. hand compartment syndrome as a result of intravenous contrast extravasation. Oxf med case rep. 2018;2018(12):omy098 [8]).

3. High pressure injection injuries (**Figure 3**),

4. Iatrogenic: arterial injury, reperfusion surgery, intravenous material extravasation (**Figure 4**),

5. Infection: abscess, septic tenosynovitis, necrotizing fasciitis,

6. Bites (snake, insect),

7. Anticoagulation medications,

8. muscle overuse (exercise, tetany, seizures) [4, 8, 13, 14].

4. Diagnosis

Patient's history, clinical image and physical examination are the keystones for the diagnosis of acute compartment syndrome [2]. Localized swelling and disproportionate pain, unresponsive to analgesics, along with a relative mechanism of injury should raise the suspicion of ACS [2, 4, 13]. As mentioned in the anatomy section, sensory nerves of the hand are located outside the compartments, with the exception of the median and digital nerves. Hence, tingling and paresthesia are not always present, unless the carpal tunnel or digits are involved [4, 5].

Serial clinical examination is of paramount importance, in order to detect ACS early. On inspection, severe swelling is noticed. Blisters might also be visible. The hand is sitting in intrinsic minus position, i.e. the metacarpophalangeal joints (MCPJs) are in extension and the interphalangeal joints (IPJs) are in slight flexion (**Figure 4**) [1, 4, 8]. Digital palpation reveals great tension of the hand. Pain on passive stretching of the intracompartmental muscles is an early sign of impaired blood perfusion. Specifically for the hand, each compartment should be stretched individually. The interossei compartments are stretched by passively abducting and adducting the digits and at the same time keeping the MCPJs in flexion and the IPJs in extension (bring the hand from the intrinsic minus position to the intrinsic plus position - "intrinsic stretch test"). The lumbricals are stretched by passively extending the MCPJ and flexing the proximal IPJ. The adductor pollicis is checked by passively abducting the thumb. Passive adduction of the thumb is used to test the thenar compartment and finally the hypothenar compartment is evaluated by passive adduction and extension of the small finger [2, 13]. In case the five P's of tissue ischemia are already present (pain, pallor, pulselessness, paresthesia and paralysis), then the diagnosis is considered delayed and irreversible muscle damage is very likely. Clinical examination has high specificity as well as high negative predictive value, meaning that it can exclude ACS better than confirming it [15].

In case there is any doubt regarding the diagnosis of ACS after clinical examination, or for unconscious patients, more subjective tools for evaluation should be used. Intracompartmental pressure measurement (ICP) is considered to be the main adjunct to the diagnosis. It is generally accepted that a pressure difference (ΔP) between the diastolic blood pressure (Pd) and the compartmental pressure (Pc) less than 30 mmHg necessitates surgical decompression ($\Delta P = Pd - Pc < 30$ mmHg). This difference is more reliable than an absolute intracompartmental pressure of more than 30 mmHg [15, 16]. Several modalities of measuring the pressure of the compartments have been described, such as the infusion Whiteside apparatus, the slit catheter technique and the handheld intracompartmental pressure monitoring [13]. Straight catheters have the least accuracy as compared to the slit catheter and side port needle. It is also reported that the Whiteside apparatus overestimates the intracompartmental pressure, which can potentially lead to an unnecessary fasciotomy [2, 15]. Current trend is towards a continuous pressure measurement, which is probably more reliable than a single one, as the latter approach is associated with a high false positive rate [17, 18]. As there are cases of silent compartment syndrome described in the literature, i.e. severe swelling with no excruciating pain, whenever there is a slight suspicion of ACS, ICP measurement should be performed [18].

Regardless of the apparatus used, it is crucial that a correct technique of pressure measurement is performed. General guidelines include perpendicular insertion of the needle on the skin [2], within 5 cm of the fracture site, but not in direct contact with the fracture [15, 16]. Particularly for the hand, each compartment's pressure should be measured individually. The hand should rest at the level of the heart. For the thenar and hypothenar compartment the needle is inserted at the border of glabrous and nonglabrous skin. The adductor pollicis muscle is entered ulnarly to the first metacarpal. The interossei compartments are entered between the index-long, long-ring and ring-small finger metacarpal, 1 cm proximal to the metacarpal heads, superficial at first for the dorsal interrosei muscle and then 0,5 to 1 cm deeper for the volar interrosei. Needle insertion over the midpalmar lesion is also used for carpal tunnel pressure measurement (**Figure 5**) [2, 4].

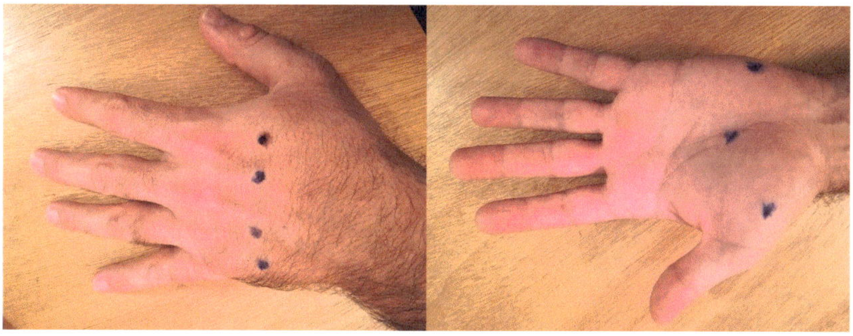

Figure 5.
Portals of intracompartmental pressure measurement of the hand.

Given the fact that clinical examination and intracompartmental pressure measurements have their own limitations, recent research is directed towards hemodynamic and metabolic parameters in an effort to achieve a more accurate diagnosis of ACS. These parameters include: a. Monitoring local oxygenation (via intramuscular partial oxygen pressure, oxygen saturation measurement or near infrared spectroscopy), b. monitoring local perfusion (via pulsed phased - locked loop ultrasound, photoplethysmography, laser Doppler flowmetry and scintigraphy), c. local metabolic analysis (intramuscular glucose monitoring, intramuscular pH monitoring) and d. serum biomarkers (white blood cell count, erythrocyte sedimentation rate, C - reative protein and creatinine kinase). However there is still no evidence of superiority over intracompartmental pressure measurement and there is still long way to go until they can be used safely in clinical practise [16].

Chronic exertional compartment syndrome is defined as a muscle dysfunction because of ICP rising due to excessive activity. Only few cases of chronic compartment syndrome located in the hand have been described in the literature and the most commonly affected compartments are the adductor pollicis, the first dorsal interosseous, the thenar and hypothenar compartments [19].

5. Treatment

Muscles can tolerate a condition of reduced vascular supply for a time period of no more than 6 to 8 hours. Regarding the limbs there is evidence supporting that the time threshold after which necrosis occurs, is 8 hours [6]. There are though case series reporting a good outcome from fasciotomies which were performed within 12 hours [11]. Impeded compartment syndrome should be recognized early, in order to avoid loss of limb function. Once the diagnosis is made, every effort should be done to decrease the intracompartmental pressure. Conservative treatment includes simple releasing of dressings or splitting a tight cast. The hand should be elevated at the level of the heart, but not above it, in order to preserve the arterio-venous gradient. Oxygen supplementation, intravenous hydration and mannitol adminstration are additional adjuvants to operative treatment [10]. Surgical decompression through fasciotomies is the mainstay of treatment, if acute compartment syndrome is suspected [3, 13].

Faciotomies of the hand are performed through four skin incision. a. Two dorsal incisions over the second and the fourth metacarpal are recommended for decompression of the interossei's and adductor pollicis' compartments. Blunt dissection is carried out deeper through the fascia between the 1st dorsal interossei and the adductor pollicis and between the dorsal and palmar interossei muscles. b. One incision radial to the first metacarpal between the glabrous and nonglabrous skin for the thenar decompression. c. One incision ulnar to the fifth metacarpal for the hypothenar release. d. Carpal tunnel, although not a true compartment, it should be released through the traditional midpalmar longitudinal incision (**Figure 6**) [2–4]. e. If digits

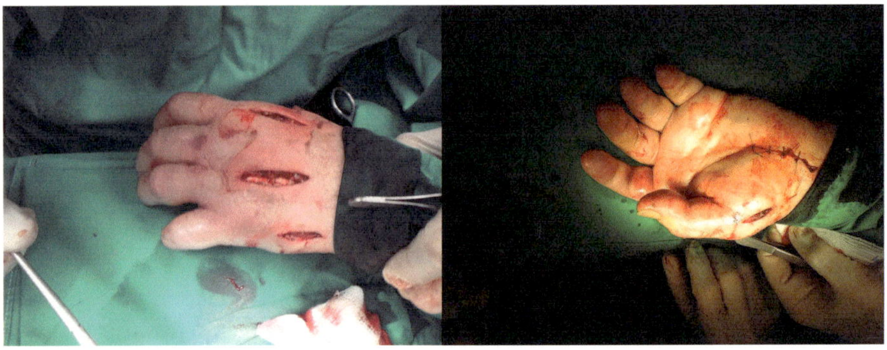

Figure 6.
Hand fasciotomies. Two dorsal incisions over the second and fourth metacarpal are used to decompress the adductor pollicis and interossei compartments. One incision radial and palmar to the first metacarpal for the thenar compartment. One incision ulnar to the fifth metacarpal for the hypothenar compartment. One midpalmar incision for carpal tunnel release. (from: Stavrakakis IM et al. hand compartment syndrome as a result of intravenous contrast extravasation. Oxf med case rep. 2018;2018(12):omy098 [8]).

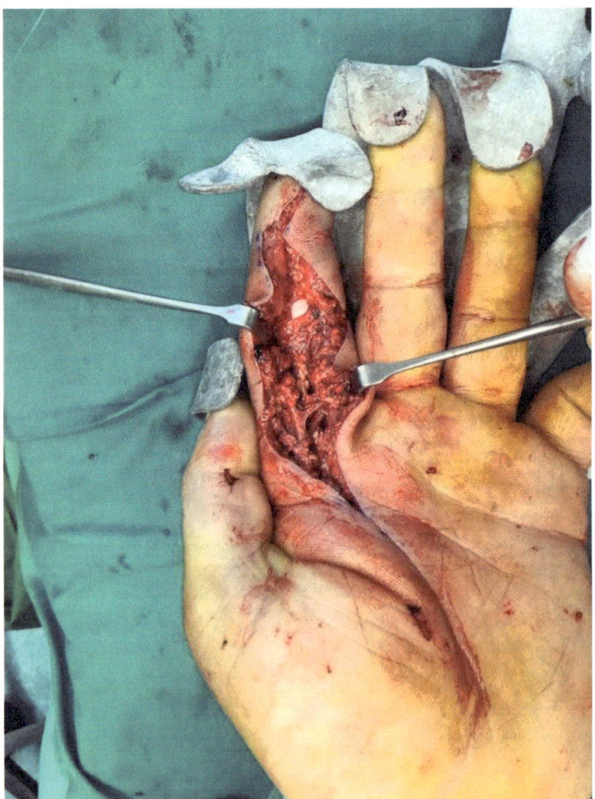

Figure 7.
Surgical decompression of index finger's compartment syndrome, due to high pressure injection injury, complicated with septic tenosynovitis of the patient of the ***Figure 3****. Proper debridement required a volar Brunner incision instead of a lateral one, which is normally used for digital compartment syndrome.*

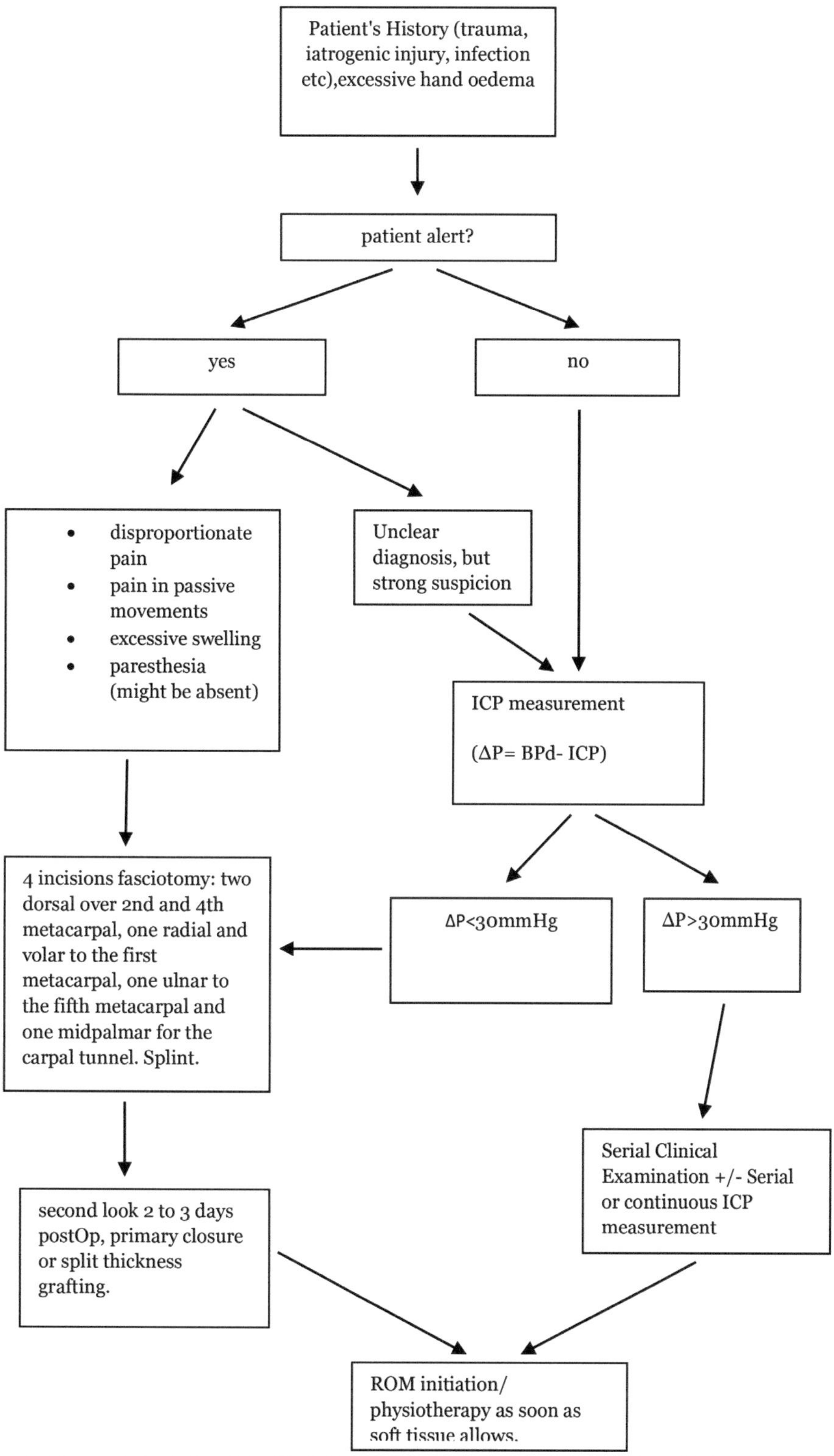

Table 2.
Algorithm of hand ACS management. ΔP: pressure difference, BPd: diastolic blood pressure, ICP: intracompartmental pressure.

are involved, Cleland and Grayson ligaments are released through midaxial lateral incision, 4 cm long centered over the proximal interphallangeal joint (PIPJ), taking care of the neurovascular bundle. Dominant sensory nerves should be avoided, indicating a radial incision for the thumb and the small finger and ulnar incision for the index, middle and ring fingers [2, 13]. In delayed cases though, especially if they are complicated with infection, a volar Brunner incision is suggested (**Figure 7**). After the procedure, the wounds are generally left opened and the hand is splinted in a safe position of function. In case of severe skin damage (burns), which precludes the splint application, the metacarpophallangeal (MTPJ) joints are pinned in flexion and the PIPJs in extension (intrinsic plus position) [2, 4]. The wounds are inspected every 2 to 3 days and a second debridement is suggested, if signs of infection or necrosis are identified. As soon as edema subsides and circulation is restored, the wounds can either be closed primarily or they can receive a split thickness graft. Priority is given to the coverage of tendons and nerves. Physiotherapy is initiated as early as possible [2, 10]. Proposed treatment algorithm of acute hand compartment syndrome is presented on the **Table 2**.

A good functional outcome can be expected after ACS, if surgical release is performed early. In case of a neglected compartment syndrome, it is widely accepted that delayed fasciotomies (more than 24 hours since initial presentation), are no beneficial to the patient, and they actually carry a risk of serious complications, such as infection, septicemia and amputation. Fasciotomies are also associated with stiffness, pain, cosmetic problems, nerve injury and chronic venous insufficiency [15, 16]. If the hand compartment syndrome is not managed properly, permanent loss of function is inevitable. Muscle contractures are developed and the hand sits in intrinsic minus position, with the MCPJs in extension and the PIPJs in flexion. Intrinsic plus contraction though is possible, if lumbricals muscles are predominantly affected. The first web space is contracted as well [2, 20].

Hand ischaemic contractures includes three groups. Group 1: All interrosei and thenar muscles are involved (typical Volkmann contracture). Group 2: thenar or interossei muscles are involved. Deformity concerns the thumb or the fingers. Group 3: one or more fingers are affected. Established intrinsic muscles contractures are treated with appropriate operative releases. The first web space is released and the tendons of the interossei muscles are released at the level of the metacarpal necks. Fibrotic tissue is removed. Detailed description of these operations are beyond the scope of this chapter [20, 21].

6. Conclusion

Hand compartment syndrome is an urgent condition which demands early recognition and treatment, otherwise it results to a permanent loss of function. Several controversies regarding diagnosis and management still exist in the contemporary literature. Future research should target on how a more accurate and early diagnosis can be achieved and the time frame beyond which fasciotomy is not beneficial to the patient. Fasciotomies of the hand are the cornerstone of treatment, and if they are performed early, they guarantee a good functional outcome. The surgeon should demonstrate a low threshold towards surgical release if compartment syndrome is suspected. Knowledge of the special anatomical features of the hand is necessary, in order for the physician to offer to the patient a sufficient treatment.

Author details

Ioannis M. Stavrakakis[1*], George E. Magarakis[1] and Theodoros H. Tosounidis[2]

1 Venizeleio General Hospital of Heraklion Crete, Greece

2 Medical School, University of Crete, Greece

*Address all correspondence to: i.m.stavrakakis@gmail.com

References

[1] Seiler III JG, Olvey SP. Compartment syndromes of the hand and forearm. J Am Soc Surg Hand. 2003;3(4):184-198. doi:10.1016/S1531-0914(03)00072-X

[2] Rubinstein AJ, Ahmed IH, Vosbikian MM. Hand compartment syndrome. Hand Clin. 2018;34(1):41-52. doi: 10.1016/j.hcl.2017.09.005

[3] Codding JL, Vosbikian MM, Ilyas AM. Acute compartment syndrome of the hand. J Hand Surg. 2015;40(6):1213-1216. doi: 10.1016/j.jhsa.2015.01.034

[4] Oak NR, Abrams RA. Compartment syndrome of the hand. Orthop Clin. 2016;47(3):609-616. doi: 10.1016/j.ocl.2016.03.006

[5] Reichman EF. Compartment Syndrome of the Hand: a little thought about diagnosis. Case Rep Emerg Med. 2016;2016. doi: 10.1155/2016/2907067

[6] Coccolini F, Improta M, Picetti E, Vergano LB, Catena F, de'Angelis N, et al. Timing of surgical intervention for compartment syndrome in different body region: systematic review of the literature. World J Emerg Surg. 2020;15(1):1-13. doi: 10.1186/s13017-020-00339-8

[7] DiFelice Jr A, Seiler III JG, Whitesides Jr TE. The compartments of the hand: an anatomic study. J Hand Surg. 1998;23(4):682-686. doi: 10.1016/S0363-5023(98)80055-5

[8] Stavrakakis IM, Daskalakis II, Detsis EPS, Karagianni CA, Papantonaki SN, Katsafarou MS. Hand compartment syndrome as a result of intravenous contrast extravasation. Oxf Med Case Rep. 2018;2018(12):omy098. doi: 10.1093/omcr/omy098

[9] Guyton G, Shearman C, Saltzman C. Compartmental divisions of the hand revisited: rethinking the validity of cadaver infusion experiments. J Bone Joint Surg Br. 2001;83(2):241-244. doi: 10.1302/0301-620X.83B2.0830241

[10] Mabvuure NT, Malahias M, Hindocha S, Khan W, Juma A. Acute Compartment Syndrome of the Limbs: Current Concepts and Management. Open Orthop J. 2012;6:535. doi: 10.2174/1874325001206010535

[11] Garner MR, Taylor SA, Gausden E, Lyden JP. Compartment syndrome: diagnosis, management, and unique concerns in the twenty-first century. HSS Journal®. 2014;10(2):143-152. doi: 10.1007/s11420-014-9386-8

[12] Heppenstall RB, Sapega AA, Scott R, Shenton D, Park YS, Maris J, et al. The compartment syndrome: an experimental and clinical study of muscular energy metabolism using phosphorus nuclear magnetic resonance spectroscopy. Clin Orthop Relat Res. 1988;226:138-55. PMID: **3275510**

[13] Chandraprakasam T, Kumar RA. Acute compartment syndrome of forearm and hand. Indian J Plast Surg. 2011;44(2). doi: 10.4103/0970-0358.85342

[14] Selek H, Özer H, Aygencel G, Turanlı S. Compartment syndrome in the hand due to extravasation of contrast material. Arch Orthop Trauma Surg. 2007;127(6):425-427. doi: 10.1007/s00402-006-0238-y

[15] Guo J, Yin Y, Jin L, Zhang R, Hou Z, Zhang Y. Acute compartment syndrome: Cause, diagnosis, and new viewpoint. Medicine (Baltimore). 2019;98(27). doi: 10.1097/MD.0000000000016260

[16] McMillan TE, Gardner WT, Schmidt AH, Johnstone AJ. Diagnosing acute compartment syndrome—where

have we got to? Int Orthop. 2019;1-7. doi: 10.1007/s00264-019-04386-y

[17] McQueen MM, Duckworth AD, Aitken SA. The estimated sensitivity and specificity of compartment pressure monitoring for acute compartment syndrome. JBJS. 2013;95(8):673-677. doi: 10.2106/JBJS.K.01731.

[18] Badhe S, Baiju D, Elliot R, Rowles J, Calthorpe D. The 'silent'compartment syndrome. Injury. 2009;40(2):220-2. doi: 10.1016/j.injury.2008.07.023

[19] Dwyer CL, Soong MC, Kasparyan NG. Chronic exertional compartment syndrome of the hand: case report and literature review. Hand. 2017;12(3):NP43–NP45. doi: 10.1177/1558944716668826

[20] McLardy-Smith, P., P. D. Burge, and N. A. Watson. "Ischaemic contracture of the intrinsic muscles of the hands a Hazard of physical restraint." The Journal of Hand Surgery: British & European Volume 11.1 (1986): 65-67.

[21] Balakrishnan G. CME-Ischaemic contracture of the hand. Indian J Plast Surg. 2006;39(1):94-102.

Section 3

Compartment Syndrome in Extramusculoskeletal Sites

Chapter 3

Thoracoabdominal Compartment Syndrome

Abdulaziz Shaher

Abstract

As we advance our knowledge in understanding abdominal compartment syndrome, it is worth going back to revisit our basic embryologic development of the main determinant of the abdominal and thoracic cavities, i.e., the diaphragm. The abdominal and thoracic cavities used to be one cavity at some stage of the embryonic life — "intraembryonic coelom" — before the "septum transversum" — diaphragmatic origin — divided it into two cavities. Therefore, if a condition develops that will impair the diaphragm from separating the cavities, leading to the possibility of pressures to transmit from one cavity to another, this becomes relevant as abdominal compartment syndrome. Diaphragmatic eventration is a congenital developmental defect in the muscular portion of the diaphragm with preserved attachments to the sternum, ribs, and dorsolumbar spine, leading to a semi-membranous diaphragm that anatomically separates the two cavities, but not physiologically. In the case of high abdominal pressure, the pressure will transmit to the thoracic cavity, causing derangement in both the anatomy and physiology. This was reported and named "Thoracoabdominal Compartment Syndrome".

Keywords: Thoracoabdominal Compartment Syndrome, eventration, diaphragmatic paralysis, abdominal compartment syndrome

1. Introduction

The diaphragm is formed from a number of composite origins in the embryo. The most important is the "septum transversum", which is a thick mass of cranial mesenchyme that gives rise to parts of the thoracic diaphragm. Without dwelling into more details, the septum transversum merges with mesoderm surrounding the esophagus, the growing pleura and peritoneum ('pleuroperitoneal folds') and the growing muscles of the abdominal wall. The septum transversum gives rise to the central tendon, while the pleuroperitoneal fold and abdominal wall muscles give rise to the muscular posterolateral parts.

Figures 1 and **2** show a brief introduction on the embryogenic development of the diaphragm and the truncal cavities.

The incidence of fetal breathing increases at up to about 30 weeks of gestation. Once the fetal breathing movements are characterized by a fluent downward movement of the diaphragm, outward displacement of the abdomen and inward displacement of the thorax occur [1].

After birth, the movement of the diaphragm accounts for the majority of the change in intrathoracic volume during quiet inspiration until it reaches 75% in adulthood. The diaphragmatic fibers attach around the inferior aspect of the

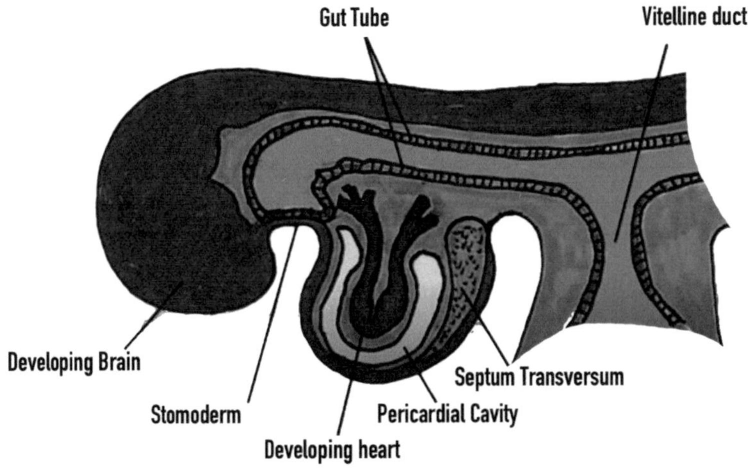

Figure 1.
Sagittal View of the embryo at 8 weeks, showing the early development of septum transversum.

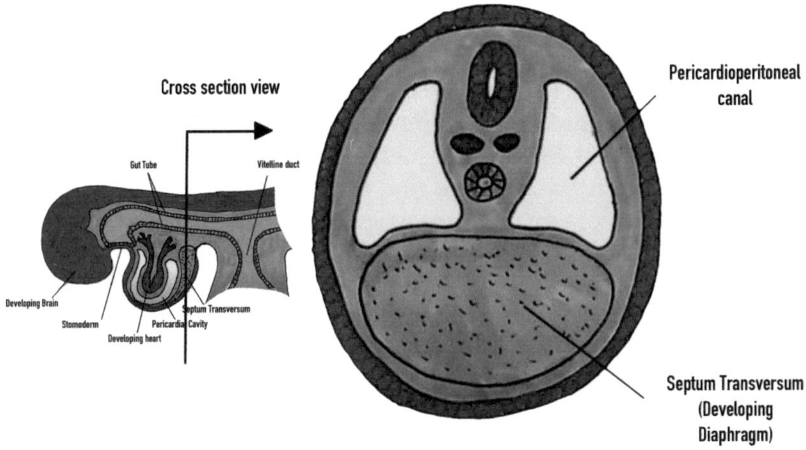

Figure 2.
Cross sectional view at the level of the septum transversum (Drawn by the author).

thoracic cage, arching over the liver and contracting downward (inspiration) and relaxing upwards (expiration), exactly like a piston. The movement distance can be up to 7 cm with deep inspiration, and as a result, it is the main determinant of abdominal pressure, along with the abdominal wall muscles and fat [2].

For example, during vomiting and eructation, intra-abdominal pressure is increased by contraction of the costal fibers, but the crural fibers remain relaxed, allowing material to pass from the stomach into the esophagus [2].

The maximum transdiaphragmatic pressure (Pdimax) reflects the diaphragmatic function and force. To measure Pdimax (the difference between intra-abdominal and intrathoracic pressures), pressure transducers are placed through the external nares to the stomach (to approximate intra-abdominal pressure) and in the esophagus (to approximate intrathoracic pressure). However, this technique is not commonly utilized.

Measuring pleural pressure is essential in ventilated patients in the Intensive Care Unit who have Acute Respiratory Distress Syndrome (ARDS). Accurate measurement of the ventilator parameters is required to assure safe and effective ventilation for already injured lungs.

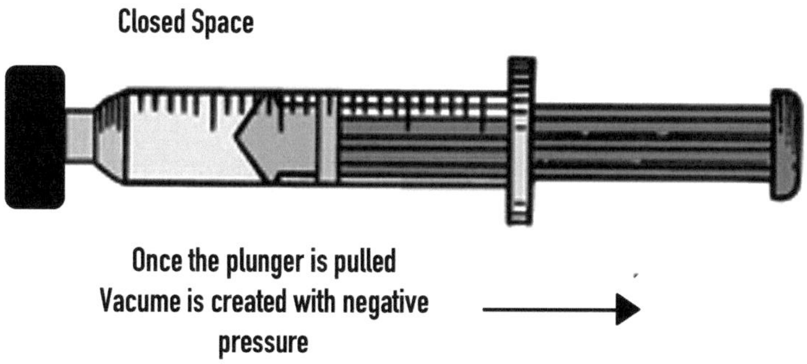

Figure 3.
Creating the negative pressure by syringe plunger simulating the action of the diaphragm.

The diaphragm behaves very much like the plunger of a syringe; inspiration contracts the diaphragmatic fibers, pulling the diaphragm downwards and decreasing the pressure (negative value below atmospheric pressure) in the thoracic cavity. This activity allows air to flow to the chest (**Figure 3**).

2. Diaphragmatic eventration

Diaphragmatic eventration is an uncommon condition that is usually incidentally discovered. The classical patient presentation is an incidental elevation hemidiaphragm on chest X-ray. The most important and common imitator of eventration is diaphragmatic paralysis, which has a different etiology and histopathological picture; however, the clinical presentation in adults is similar and these two conditions are sometimes very difficult to distinguish from each other.

True diaphragmatic eventration is a congenital developmental defect in the muscular portion of the diaphragm with preserved attachments to the sternum, ribs, and dorsolumbar spine, maintaining the anatomical separation of the two cavities. It is rare, with an incidence of <0.05%, more common in males, and more often affects the left hemidiaphragm [3].

In contrast to true diaphragmatic eventration, diaphragmatic paralysis is a more common, acquired condition that generally results from traumatic or iatrogenic injury to the phrenic nerve or as a result of tumor invasion.

Diaphragmatic eventration can be bilateral, unilateral, or localized to a certain anatomical zone of the diaphragm (anterior, posterolateral, or medial) [3]. Microscopically, the eventrated portion has disseminated fibroelastic tissues at the expense of myocytes [4]. Patients with diaphragmatic paralysis have a normal amount of muscle fibers, but the main issue is their atrophy.

There have been multiple descriptions of associations of diaphragmatic eventration with other congenital abnormalities like dextrocardia, intestinal malrotation and renal agenesis [5].

Patients who have diaphragmatic eventration may not have the normal caudal movement of the diaphragm necessary for appropriate inspiration. As a result, diaphragmatic movement can be diminished, absent, or even paradoxic.

An imaging study required to diagnose eventration besides chest X-ray is fluoroscopy. Specifically, a fluoroscopic sniff test is indicated. During this test, the diaphragm normally moves downward during sniffing; however, in paralysis or eventration, it moves upwards.

The main treatment for eventrated diaphragm is diaphragmatic plication through various either open or minimally invasive. While diaphragmatic pacing is mainly quadriplegics with diaphragmatic paralysis.

3. Syndromes with increased truncal compartmental pressures

3.1 Tension pneumothorax

Tension pneumothorax is a well-known pathophysiological state in which the thoracic cavity develops very high pressure as a result of accumulated air in the pleural cavity, displacing the mediastinum and preventing the preload from draining back to the right side of the heart. This can affect left-sided heart afterload and ultimately lead to hemodynamic compromise.

The most common mechanism is traumatic lung injury, or iatrogenic injury due central venous cannulation. According to the American Trauma Life Support manual [6], the management of such a life-threatening injury is immediate pleural decompression. This can be done in many ways depending on the physician's experience; either by using a needle, finger, or intercostal pleural drainage tube, as long it is done promptly and safely, to not cause any further injuries. Once the drainage is done, the tension pneumothorax will turn into a simple pneumothorax and the management of a simple pneumothorax is beyond the scope of this book.

3.2 Tension pneumoperitoneum and ascites (Hydroperitoneum)

Tension pneumoperitoneum is a much less known pathology compared to tension pneumothorax [7]. In this condition, air or fluid accumulates in the peritoneal cavity, leading to respiratory and hemodynamic compromise. The most common cause of pneumoperitoneum is pathological perforated viscus (e.g., perforated duodenal ulcers, perforated colonic mass). Peritoneal fluid can increase in the abdomen in large amounts, reaching 10–15 L (ascites or hydroperitoneum) due to advanced liver cirrhosis, or it can be malignant ascites secondary to advanced metastatic abdominal malignancy. Both of these conditions can lead to increases in abdominal pressure and compromise of respiratory function.

As a result of increasing cases of liver cirrhosis worldwide, the incidence of cirrhosis-induced ascites is common, and the effect of massive ascites on respiratory function and thoracoabdominal movement (cirtometry) have been studied before and after paracentesis [8]. After paracentesis, minute ventilation, tidal volume, and dyspnea scale were better and a significant p-value, compared to before the procedure, indicated that abdominal pressure will still transmit to the pleural pressure, even in the presence of a normal diaphragm.

The term "tension" has been linked to hemodynamic compromise and shock. Therefore, for ascites to cause respiratory embarrassment without shock would not make it "tension hydroperitoneum" in the conventional wisdom. Most of the cases of hydroperitoneum and respiratory compromise reported in the literature occurred in the pediatric age group, and due to delayed perforated viscus, respiratory compromise can be explained due to the septic inflammatory response, rather than the mere machinal displacement of the diaphragm and pressure transmission [9].

The pathophysiological cascade in tension pneumoperitoneum happens at the beginning, when abdominal pressure exceeds venous pressure and the lower venous return cannot be drained back to the right side of the heart. While the upper body venous return is not enough to sustain the preload due to severe hypovolemia, this results in hemodynamic compromise, a condition termed "tension

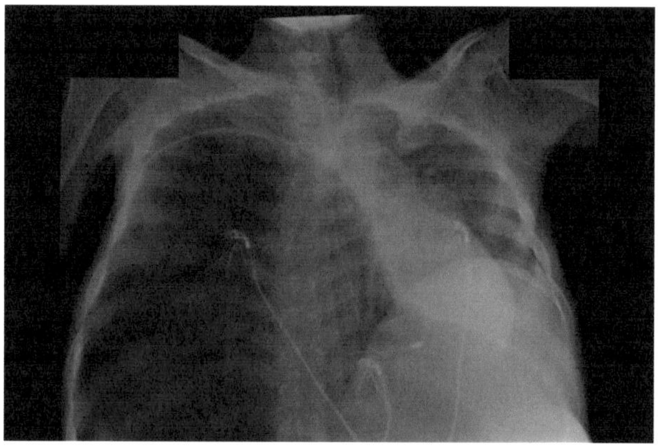

Figure 4.
Thoracoabdominal Compartment syndrome chest radiograph [11].

pneumoperitoneum". It is imperative to keep in mind that the thoracic cavity pressure should be normal because the barrier (diaphragm) should be functioning well.

What would happen if the abdominal pressure gets very high while the diaphragm is diseased and cannot prevent the pressure from transmitting to the thoracic cavity, as in diaphragmatic eventration? This condition is known as thoracoabdominal compartment syndrome.

3.3 Thoracoabdominal compartment syndrome

Thoracoabdominal compartment syndrome is a recently described syndrome, and there are a few existing case reports that describe it.

The first possible description of such a pathophysiological phenomenon was given by Haldane et al. [10], who reported a case of tension pneumoperitoneum causing hemodynamic compromise. These authors described the reason as tension pneumothorax despite the lack of air in the pleural cavity. Therefore, the exact pathophysiological association of the hemodynamic compromise, as a result of transmitted pressure from the abdominal cavity to the pleural cavity through the intact (but pliable) diaphragm, was not coined as a syndrome until Shaher et al. described it [11].

In the former report, the case was of a perforated gastric ulcer that caused tension pneumoperitoneum. The association of diaphragmatic eventration allowed an increase in abdominal pressure to be transmitted to the thoracic cavity.

The reasons for elevated abdominal pressure in this case was a significantly dilated megacolon with compromise of the thoracic cavity pressure due to the pliable diaphragm, as depicted in **Figure 4**.

A postmortem case report was recently published [12], reporting a thoracoabdominal compartment syndrome in a 65-year-old male, with the colon in right hemithorax with near total lung collapse, mediastinal shift and associated diaphragmatic eventration.

4. Conclusion

Thoracoabdominal Syndrome is a rare complication of diaphragmatic eventration, usually present with hemodynamic compromise as a result of transmitted pressure from the abdominal cavity to the pleural space. Moreover, it is usually associated with multiple congenital abnormalities. Most of the cases reported presented late due to the inability to diagnose early, leading to a very high mortality rate. Diaphragmatic eventration should be surgically repaired through plication as soon as feasible to maintain the physiological function of the diaphragm and to prevent such a syndrome from developing.

Conflict of interest

The author declares no conflicts of interest.

Author details

Abdulaziz Shaher
Armed Forces Hospital – Southern Region, Abha, Kingdom of Saudi Arabia

*Address all correspondence to: dr.shaher@gmail.com

References

[1] Dewbury K. Ultrasound in obstetrics and gynaecology. London: Churchill Livingstone; 2001.

[2] Barrett K. Ganong's review of medical physiology. New York: McGraw-Hill Education; 2019.

[3] Groth S, Andrade R. Diaphragmatic Eventration. Thoracic Surgery Clinics. 2009;19(4):511-519.

[4] Shah-Mirany J. Eventration of the Diaphragm. Archives of Surgery. 1968;96(5):844.

[5] Sharma S, Debnath P, Tripathi R. Bilateral eventration of the diaphragm with malrotation and unilateral renal agenesis. The Indian Journal of Pediatrics. 2007;74(5):503-504.

[6] Advanced Trauma Life Support. München: Elsevier, Urban et Fischer; 2015.

[7] De Smet R, De Paepe P, Buylaert W, Hachimi Idrissi S. Spontaneous tension pneumoperitoneum presenting as an out of hospital cardiac arrest: A case report and review of the literature. Acta Clinica Belgica. 2016;71(4):258-262.

[8] Witter V, Lima R, Maia M, Duarte H, Paro F. Respiratory and symptomatic impact of ascites relief by paracentesis in patients with hepatic cirrhosis. Arquivos de Gastroenterologia. 2020;57(1):64-68.

[9] Im S, Lim G, Hahn S. Spontaneous gastric perforation in a neonate presenting with massive hydroperitoneum. Pediatric Radiology. 2005;35(12):1212-1214.

[10] Akoglu H, Coban E, Guneysel O. Tension pneumoperitoneum complicated with tension pneumothorax in a patient with diaphragmatic eventration. Case Reports. 2012;2012(apr04 1): bcr0120125512-bcr0120125512.

[11] Shaher A, Alqahtani AM, Sinnah KN, Al Bakheet SM. Diaphragmatic eventration unusual presentation: A novel thoracoabdominal compartment syndrome case. BMJ Case Rep. 2019;12(6):e229475.

[12] Omenai SA, Adebowale EO, Nwanji ID. Thoracoabdominal compartment syndrome complicating right-sided diaphragmatic eventration with co-existent unilateral renal agenesis. Autops Case Rep [Internet]. 2020;10(2):e2020155.

Chapter 4

Abdominal Compartment Syndrome

Kuo-Ching Yuan, Chih-Yuan Fu and Hung-Chang Huang

Abstract

Abdominal compartment syndrome (ACS) is a progressively increasing intraabdominal pressure of more than 20 mm Hg with new-onset thoracoabdominal organ dysfunction. Primary abdominal compartment syndrome means increased pressure due to injury or disease in the abdominopelvic region. Secondary abdominal compartment syndrome means disease originating from outside the abdomen, such as significant burns or sepsis. As the pressure inside the abdomen increases, organ failure occurs, and the kidneys and lungs are the most frequently affected. Managements of ACS are multidisciplinary. Conservative treatment with adequate volume supple and with aggressive hemodynamic support is the first step. Decompressive laparotomy with open abdomen is indicated when ACS is refractory to conservative treatment and complicated with multiple organ failure. ACS can result in a high mortality rate, and successful treatment requires cooperation between physicians, intensivists, and surgeons.

Keywords: abdominal compartment syndrome, intraabdominal pressure, intensive care unit, open abdomen, multiple organ failure

1. Introduction

A compartment syndrome happened when the pressure in a closed anatomic space increases to a level that compromises surrounding tissue viability. In the abdominal space with elevated pressure, the impact to the end-organ function within and outside the abdominal cavity can be lethal. The abdominal compartment syndrome (ACS) is not a solo disease; it can have many causes and develop many disease processes. ACS is a highly under-recognized but very lethal entity [1–3]. If inadequately treated, the patient may rapidly proceed into multiple organ failure, and patient mortality. In a systemic review, the reported prevalence of Intra-Abdominal Hypertension (IAH) and ACS is about 30% to 49% [4]. The prevalence is exceptionally high in pancreatitis (57%), orthotopic liver transplantation (7%), and abdominal aorta surgery (5%) [5]. It is reported that Body mass index (odds ratio 1.08, 95% confidence interval 1.03–1.13), mechanical ventilation (OR 3.52, 95% CI 2.08–5.96), and APACHE IV score at ICU admission (OR 1.03, 95% CI 1.02–1.04) are risk factors for IAH or ACS occurrence [5].

ACS has received heightened attention in critical care medicine, and the prevention of IAH and ACS are of tremendous importance in the care of critically ill, surgical, and trauma patients. The etiology of ACS is various and can be complicated. Diagnosis is made by clinical presentations and intraabdominal pressure (IAP) measurements. Serial or continuous IAP measurements are essential to the timely diagnosis, proper management, and good recovery in these patients. Urinary bladder pressure measurement is an excellent method to estimate for IAP as it is easily performed in all patients at risk for significant elevations in IAP [6–8]. A pressure more than 12 mmHg is considered IAH, and if the IAP is higher than 20 mmHg with new-onset organ failure, it is ACS. Medical treatment is usually adopted first, and decompressive laparotomy is indicated if medical treatment failed. The development of ACS can profoundly impact patient recovery and outcome. The rate of renal replacement therapy was much higher in ACS (38.9%) than in patients with normal intra-abdominal pressure (1.2%). Both intensive care and 90-day mortality were also significantly higher in ACS (16.7% and 38.9%) than regular IAP patients (1.2% and 7.1%) [5].

2. Pathophysiology

The abdomen is in anatomy a closed space with surrounding structures either rigid (costal arch, spine, and pelvis) or elastic (the muscular wall and diaphragm). The elasticity of the walls and the parenchymal character of abdominal contents determine the pressure inside the abdomen. Most of the abdomen contents are essentially non-compressive and behavior as fluid by Pascal's law; the pressure detected at any point can represent the pressure within the whole abdomen [9]. IAP is literally a status with steady pressure within a conceal cavity, and the reference range is approximately 5–7 mmHg and is increasing to 12–15 mmHg postoperatively. Diseases associated with a chronic elevated IAP include ascites after liver cirrhosis, ovarian tumors, chronic ambulatory peritoneal dialysis (CAPD), and obesity.

IAP that is more than 12 mm Hg is intra-abdominal hypertension (IAH) and has four grades [1]:

- grade I: 12–15 mmHg
- grade II: 16–20 mmHg
- grade III: 21–25 mmHg
- grade IV: > 25 mm Hg

The WSACS proposed the following classification for IAH [1]: Primary IAH results from injury or disease from the abdominal-pelvis requiring surgical or other intervention. Secondary IAH is the result due to disease not associated with the abdominopelvic disease. Recurrent IAH is the condition redeveloped following previous management of primary or secondary IAH/ACS.

Abdominal compartment syndrome is defined as a sustained IAP of at least 20 mm Hg associated with new organ dysfunction/failure. It should be noted that the IAP ranges associated with these grades have been revised downward in recent years as the detrimental impact of elevated IAP on end-organ function has been recognized. Physiologically, IAP increases with inspiration (diaphragmatic contraction) and decreases with expiration (diaphragmatic relaxation). Pathophysiology of ACS is multifactorial. With the increasing of pressures inside abdomen, compression of the arterial inflow at first and then compression of the venous outflow of the visceral organs can lead to organ hypoperfusion. Compression of the blood vessels also damage heart function. Besides, the diaphragm's upward displacement can lead to hypoventilation, respiratory rate changes, and eventually hypoxia [10]. This complex physiological

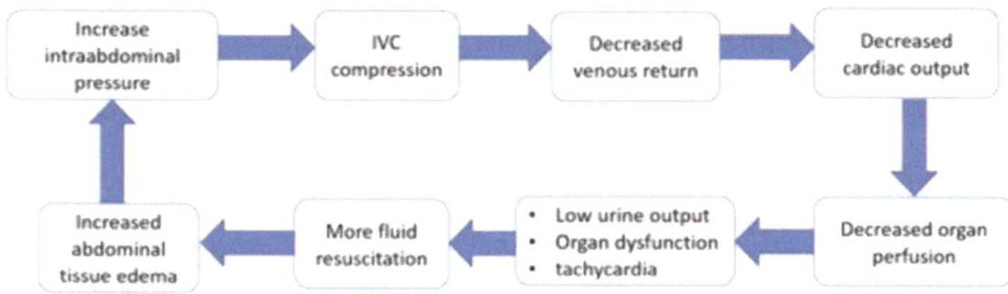

Figure 1.
Vicious cycle of elevated intraabdominal pressure.

change regarding the organ system mentioned above can be applied to all body systems concerning impact caused by ACS. Elevated IAP can lead to a vicious cycle and result in multiple organ failure (**Figure 1**). Elevated intra-abdominal pressured causes IVC compression and reduced venous return as venous return reduced, so as cardiac output reduced. Therefore, many organs suffered from low perfusion and presented with organ dysfunction as clinical signs. Aggressive fluid resuscitation may be prescribed, which leads to progressive tissue edema with increasing intraabdominal pressure.

Abdominal perfusion pressure (APP), calculated as MAP minus IAP, has been proposed as a predictor of visceral perfusion and a potential endpoint for resuscitation [11, 12]. By considering both arterial inflow (MAP) and restrictions to venous outflow (IAP), APP has been demonstrated as a parameter predicting patient survival from IAH and ACS. Studies have also identified that APP is also superior to other standard resuscitation endpoints, including arterial pH, base deficit, arterial lactate, and hourly urinary output [11]. A target APP of more than 60 mmHg is positively correlated with better survival from IAH and ACS [11].

- Definition: APP = MAP – IAP.

3. Clinical manifestation

Increased respiration rate is usually the first detected clinical sign at the initial development of ACS, even with ventilator and sedation. Although tachypnea may have resulted from hypovolemia or hemorrhage, the whole clinical presentation is not compatible with low volume status since CVP is usually high or positive fluid balance. Application of bedside echo and thorough physical exam can often detect massive ascites or hemoperitoneum. ACS is usually the consequence or complication of a particular medical disease or medical treatment. The most common cause of ACS is major abdominal trauma, abdominal sepsis, and pancreatitis. The medical treatments that can cause ACS are massive transfusion, intraperitoneal packing, and intra-aorta stent for ruptured abdominal aorta aneurysm. Primary symptoms of ACS include abdominal pain and distention. Secondary signs of ACS include respiratory depression, decreased cardiac output, visceral ischemia due to decreased perfusion, and renal failure. This condition can be fatal if not properly treated. It becomes increasingly more critical for the overall prognosis that ACS is recognized and treated timely. Detection of ACS can be interfered with by other clinical conditions. A blunt abdominal trauma patient may have active upper gastrointestinal bleeding due to stress ulcers and unstable vital signs. Hypovolemia and inadequate fluid resuscitation may be the first impression as the cause of shock. However, CT may also reveal massive hemoperitoneum compressing intra-abdominal contents leading to ACS. This kind of patient may present with hemodynamic instability as the first clinical indicator of ACS.

4. Radiographic features

Computed tomography is the most used method for etiology evaluation in patients with a distended abdomen. CT findings suggestive of ACS include a tense infiltration of the retroperitoneum exceeding primary peritoneal disease, narrowing the inferior vena cava due to external compression, and an increased ratio of anteroposterior-to-transverse abdominal diameter. Besides, compression or displacement of the kidney, extensive bowel wall thickening with enhancement, and simultaneously bilateral inguinal herniation are also potentially indicative of ACS [13].

The ratio of maximal anteroposterior to the transverse abdominal diameter and peritoneal-to-abdomen height ratio are reported statistically associated with elevated IAP [14]. There are several other signs in CT and echo that may support the diagnosis of ACS. Still, most of these are considered nonspecific or insensitive for ACS [15]. Suppose CT findings suggestive of increased intraabdominal pressure are noticed. In that case, the radiologist should swiftly communicate with physicians to treat the patient because the abdominal compartment syndrome may require urgent intervention.

5. Measuring IAP

IAP monitoring and IAH/ACS management are increasing importance as critical for the patient outcome; various pressure measurement methods using either direct (abdominal pressure measurement with a catheter) and indirect (use pressure inside the urinary bladder, stomach, colon, or uterine) techniques have been suggested [16–18]. Among these methods, the bladder technique is the most widespread adoption due to its simplicity and low cost [9, 16, 19]. Some methods providing continuous IAP measurement via the stomach, peritoneal cavity, and bladder have been validated [20–22]. The trans-bladder device can be connected with the ICU bedside monitor to provide an integrated patient monitor with other vital signs. The trans-bladder device also provides a closed system to avoid contamination and reduce urinary tract infection (**Figure 2**). Although these techniques seem promising, more clinical validation is required before general use can be recommended.

One of the questions for IAP measurement is the reference point. Many studies had suggested using the symphysis pubis is widely used in many studies as the reference point, but this can cause different IAP results within the same patient in some clinical conditions. For example, changes in different body positions (supine,

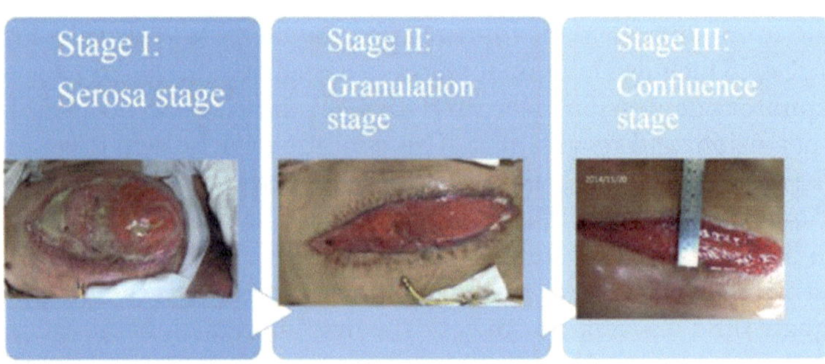

Figure 2.
Wound stage of open abdomen.

prone, the elevation of head), abdominal contracture during a seizure, and abnormal bladder detrusor muscle contractions have been demonstrated to impact the accuracy of IAP measurements [9].

Another disparity among IAP measurement techniques is the priming-volume instilled into the bladder to ensure a conductive fluid column between the bladder wall and transducer [23, 24]. Several studies have shown that too many volumes may increase bladder pressure and poorly reflect true abdominal pressure [19]. The reference standard for intermittent IAP measurement is via the bladder with a maximal installation volume of 25 ml sterile saline. Point-of-care ultrasound (POCUS) as a bedside modality in ACS patients is not well studied. A prospective observational study for patients who met the criteria of IAH was assigned to undergo POCUS and small bowel ultrasound as adjuvant tools in their IAH management [25]. POCUS can detect gastric content (fluid vs. concrete) and diagnoses of gastric paresis. POCUS can find small bowel obstruction and even mesenteric vessel occlusion or transmesenteric internal hernia. POCUS can help the nonoperative management of IAH, especially in diagnosing and treating patients with IAH.

6. Acute compartment syndrome in specific situations

6.1 ACS in post-cardiac surgery

The incidence of IAH after cardiac surgery is between 26.9% and 83.3%. There is limited evidence regarding IAH after cardiac surgery and is interpreted with caution. Obesity is a strong predictor of postoperative IAH, although not confined to a central pattern or body mass index. Prolonged cardiopulmonary bypass and aortic cross-clamp time are predisposed to IAH in some reports. IAH in cardiac surgery patients is associated with hepatic and renal failure, and corresponding biochemical markers may help screen but lack specificity. In contrast to the development of IAH in other settings, the evidence for the role of fluid balance is insufficient. Precise prediction of IAH remains challenging. Based on the present evidence, regular IAP measurement is indicated postoperatively in patients who are obese, those with preoperative renal or hepatic impairment, prolonged cardiopulmonary bypass or operative time, requiring vasopressor support, to prevent the harmful result of IAH [26].

6.2 ACS after acute pancreatitis

Acute pancreatitis can lead to severe systemic complications. ACS is one of the lethal complications of acute pancreatitis. Mortality rate in acute pancreatitis complicated with ACS can result in a 49% mortality rate, but it is only about 11% without ACS [27]. Severe form pancreatitis patients are incredibly high risk for ACS due to tissue edema after initial aggressive fluid resuscitation, profound peripancreatic inflammation, massive ascites, and ileus due to intraperitoneal inflammation. Frequent measurement of the intra-abdominal pressure is indicated for severe pancreatitis patients to obtain prompt diagnosis and treatment of ACS [28]. A high index of suspicion is needed for patient care of acute pancreatitis. Management of ACS after pancreatitis consists of supportive care and abdominal decompression if indicated. The highest mortality rate reported in patients with necrotizing pancreatitis and decompression laparotomy reduces it by 8.7%. Decompressive laparotomy should be used as soon as possible if medical resuscitation failure [29].

6.3 ACS after hip arthroplasty

A relatively rare condition is ACS after hip arthroplasty. There some case reports regarding this unusual condition [30, 31]. A patient suffered from an acetabulum fracture and received open reduction and internal fixation with hip arthroscopy. Hypothermia, increased airway pressure and oliguria happened during the operation. Desaturation and metabolic acidosis were noted. A postoperative CT revealed a large volume of irrigation fluid in the peritoneal cavity and retroperitoneum, and ACS was confirmed. The patient was treated by percutaneous peritoneal drainage and was discharged eight weeks after the operation smoothly. Intraperitoneal extravasation of irrigation fluid may occur during hip arthroscopic surgery and causes ACS later [32].

Some authors had proposed an algorithm to prevent and treat this possible lethal complication following hip arthroscopy [33].

6.4 ACS in severely burned patients

An observational study that included 56 mechanical ventilated burn patients between April 2007 and December 2009 with IAP measurement every day showed that 78.6% of patients developed IAH and 28.6% progressed into ACS [34]. Patients with ACS had larger TBSAs of burn injury (35.8 ± 30% vs. 20.6 ± 21.4%, P = 0.04) and more cumulative fluid balances after 48 hours treatment (13.6 ± 16 L vs. 7.6 ± 4.1 L, P = 0.03). The TBSA of burn injury was closely correlated with the mean IAP (R = 0.34, P = 0.01). Mortality was also significantly higher in patients with IAH (34.1% vs. 26.8%, P = 0.014) and ACS (62.5% vs. 26.8%, P < 0.0001). The author concluded that IAH/ACS incidence is high in ventilated burn patients compared to other groups of critically ill patients. The TBSA of burn injury correlates with the IAP. The combination of positive fluid balance, high IAP, elevated lung water is suggestive of an unfavorable outcome. Non-surgical interventions usually adopted for burn patient with ACS, and it appears to improve end-organ function. Since decompressive laparotomy is difficult to perform in major burn patients, the persistence of IAH is highly related to a worse outcome.

7. Treatment in ACS

As proposed by the World Society of ACS (WSACS), the standard of care is divided into two algorithms: the medical management and surgical management pathway based on clinical presentation [1]. Medical management of ACS initiated upon recognition of elevated intra-abdominal pressures (Grade I C recommendation). This includes sedation, neuromuscular blockade, evacuating intraluminal contents, paracentesis of ascites or hemoperitoneum, percutaneous drainage, cautious fluid resuscitation, and adequate organ support. The ultimate goal is an alleviation of pressures and definitive management with surgery. A protocol with serial monitoring of intra-abdominal pressures every 2–4 hours or using continuous monitoring to maintain pressures less than 15 mmHg is recommended. Percutaneous drainage is indicated in the presence of space-occupying fluid inside the peritoneal cavity. However, using catheter-directed decompression as definitive management instead of decompressive laparotomy has yet well studied.

The patient's respiratory rate, oxygenation, heart rate, and blood pressure usually rapidly improved after placing intra-abdominal catheters to alleviate the pressure. This displays the advantage of having the interventional radiology team available for definitive ACS management secondary to abdominal cavity space-occupying lesions/fluid collections. Catheter-directed drainage of ACS is indicated due to its less invasive nature and rapid availability [35]. Decompressive laparotomy may leave patients with an open abdomen with morbidities such as increased fluid losses, infection, fluid collections, fistula formation, hernias, or cosmetic concerns. Interventional radiologists are uniquely positioned to provide drainage guided management for abdominal compartment syndrome in emergent settings [36].

8. Open abdomen treatment in ACS

After decompressive laparotomy, ACS patients are usually in an open abdomen status and represent patient care difficulty. Open abdomen (OA) is a surgical technique that the abdominal fascial edges are intentionally left open after laparotomy. OA shortens the operation time and allows the patient to return to the Intensive Care Unit earlier under the unstable condition, and facilitates further treatment. OA's advantages include a concise operation time, fewer postoperative complications, and the prevention of early multiple-organ failure [37]. Besides adopted for abdominal trauma, OA is now part of the Damage-Control Surgical (DCS) for various complicated abdominal conditions, including ACS [38]. ACS usually happens in a trauma patient who received massive fluid resuscitation and blood transfusion in the primary survey and is now considered crucial to patient mortality. With the advancement in treatment regarding multiple-organ failure after trauma and ACS, decompressive laparotomy and OA patient care is now part of the essential strategy adopted to provide exemplary patient recovery.

Although the precise percentage of OA in trauma patients is not exact, this approach is now generally applied [38]. Ogilvie first reported the OA technique about 80 years ago with the design to provide adequate drainage and source control for intra-abdominal sepsis [39]. In December 2014, the first international conference for consensus about OA was held. The guidelines were proposed to clarify OA's indications, the technique for temporary abdominal closure (TAC), and the abdomen's closure. According to the Eastern Association for the Surgery of Trauma (EAST) practice management committee guidelines [40], OA is indicated when patient presented with severe metabolic acidosis (pH < 7.2), hypothermia (temperature < 35 °C), and coagulopathy, or when patient received >10 units of red blood cells transfusion, or > 6 L of crystalloids within 24 hours.

Although an open abdomen can reduce ACS mortality, it also created new problems, such as severe fluid and protein loss, nutritional problems, enter atmospheric fistulas, fascial retraction with loss of abdominal domain, and the development of massive incisional hernias [41]. A multidisciplinary approach with active interaction between the surgical team and intensive care unit team is required to manage a critically ill patient with ACS and OA, which should be done with a specific staged process with protocol [38]. A list of outlines for OA patient care is provided in **Table 1**.

Patient care challenges regarding prolonged OA include delay in extubation, the risk for repeated infections, and possible enter atmospheric fistulae. Therefore, optimizing the patient condition for the early abdomen closure is the primary goal in OA patient care. The physiological derangement of hypothermia, acidosis, and coagulopathy needs to be aggressively reversed with resuscitation in ICU. ACS patients usually have poor pulmonary compliance, and mechanical ventilation with high ventilatory pressure is necessary. We often need to cautiously distend the alveoli with high ventilatory pressure since the transpulmonary pressure is high. However, if the tidal volume is inadequate, it will cause hypoxia and respiratory

• Infection: Antibiotic use by culture result
• Nutrition: early enteral feeding
• Fluid: Maintain adequate volume status by urine amount
• Wound care: Clear gauze cover on IV bag
• Ventilation: Weaning and extubation after hemodynamic stable
• Sedation: A short duration of sedation just after operation

Table 1.
Principles for OA patient care.

acidosis, which can be fatal in an ACS patient with a tense abdomen. Once the abdomen is opened, the ventilator settings must be changed to maintain appropriate tidal volume without overexpansion of the alveoli. After OA, the increase in venous return can cause right ventricular overload if there is preexisting pulmonary hypertension due to hypercarbia or preexisting cardiomyopathy, which can be treated with dobutamine or milrinone. Significant pleural effusion may occur after OA due to increased venous load with high hydrostatic pressure, and pleural effusion drainage is indicated.

ACS patients usually have marked bowel edema, and the cause is multifactorial. The gut's perfusion is compromised during unstable blood pressure, and the mesenteric venous return is impaired when the IAP is elevated, which leads to progressive congestion in the already ischemic gut. The ischemia gut is reperfused after volume resuscitation and OA, but there is also the production of free-radical and increased mucosa permeability that can cause further bowel edema. Since a more than 10% increase in fluid-related weight gain is considered a significant negative factor for primary closure in OA [38], the goal in ICU care is to prevent fluid overload and alleviate gut edema so that a primary fascial closure can be achieved as early as possible. The OA patient can receive enteral feeding, and the only contraindication is intestinal discontinuity. Viscera exposure does not necessarily cause paralytic ileus, and feeding in OA does not cause gut edema. Early full enteral feeding should be initiated when the patient is no need to use an inotropic agent or vasopressor. Enteral feeding can maintain gut integrity, modulate the systemic inflammatory response, decrease infection rate, decrease the rate of ventilator-associated pneumonia, facilitate early closure of OA, and decrease fistulas formation. High nitrogen loss is expected in OA with ascites loss, and it is necessary to calculate the caloric demand and nitrogen balance carefully to avoid underfeeding.

Early definitive closure is the basis of preventing or reducing the risk of these complications. The key to optimizing outcome is early abdominal closure within seven days because failure to do so will increase morbidity, mortality, and fistulae formation [41, 42]. However, early fascia closure is not always feasible.

If delayed fascia closure is inevitable, proper wound care and a thorough understanding of the open abdomen is necessary. For a prolonged open abdomen, the OA wound would go through three stages (**Figure 2**). The first stage is the serosa stage, where the exposed small bowel is grossly visible, and their integrity is easily differentiated with the eyeball. In the second stage, the granulation stage, diffuse granulation tissue development over the bowel serosa happened after bowel adhesion. The outline of the small bowel is very different from the typical appearance. The third stage is the confluence stage, where the whole small bowel is in a confluent status and undifferentiable. In the third stage, the skin wound will have ingrowth into the bowel surface, and the wound will also start to contract. Therefore, the wound will become smaller and more comfortable to care for. After 3–6 months of wound care, we suggest using CT to determine the fascia gap between the open abdomen's two edges. Abdominal closure is indicated if the fascia gap is less than 8 cm.

9. Conclusion

ACS is a challenging condition in ICU patient care with a high prevalence in acute pancreatitis, orthotopic liver transplantation, and abdominal aorta surgery.

Massive resuscitation and swelling of the abdominal viscera are the primary cause of ACS. ACS can cause rapid deterioration of hemodynamic status and progresses into multiple organ failure eventually. IAP monitoring with frequent clinical evaluation is crucial for early diagnosis, and early diagnosis with prompt management is key to good patient recovery. Medical treatment is usually adopted first, but decompressive laparotomy is indicated if organ failure progresses after medical treatment. After decompressive laparotomy, the patient is in OA status, and a protocolized care plan is essential for this OA patient care.

Author details

Kuo-Ching Yuan[1]*, Chih-Yuan Fu[2] and Hung-Chang Huang[1]

1 Division of Acute Care Surgery and Trauma, Department of Surgery, Taipei Medical University Hospital, Taipei, Taiwan

2 Division of Trauma and Emergency Surgery, Department of Surgery, Chang-Gung Memorial Hospital, Linkou, Taiwan

*Address all correspondence to: traumayuan@gmail.com

References

[1] Kirkpatrick, A. W. et al. Intra-abdominal hypertension and the abdominal compartment syndrome: updated consensus definitions and clinical practice guidelines from the World Society of the Abdominal Compartment Syndrome. Intensive Care Medicine 39, 1190-1206, doi:10.1007/s00134-013-2906-z (2013).

[2] Pereira, B. M. Abdominal compartment syndrome and intra-abdominal hypertension. Current Opinion in Critical Care 25 (2019).

[3] Sosa, G., Gandham, N., Landeras, V., Calimag, A. P. & Lerma, E. Abdominal compartment syndrome. Disease-a-Month 65, 5-19, doi:https://doi.org/10.1016/j.disamonth.2018.04.003 (2019).

[4] Khot, Z. A.-O. et al. Incidence of Intra-Abdominal Hypertension and Abdominal Compartment Syndrome: A Systematic Review.

[5] Smit, M. et al. Intra-abdominal hypertension and abdominal compartment syndrome in patients admitted to the ICU. Annals of Intensive Care 10, 130, doi:10.1186/s13613-020-00746-9 (2020).

[6] Kyoung, K.-H. & Hong, S.-K. The duration of intra-abdominal hypertension strongly predicts outcomes for the critically ill surgical patients: a prospective observational study. World Journal of Emergency Surgery 10, 22, doi:10.1186/s13017-015-0016-7 (2015).

[7] Malbrain, M. L. N. G. et al. Results from the International Conference of Experts on Intra-abdominal Hypertension and Abdominal Compartment Syndrome. I. Definitions. Intensive Care Medicine 32, 1722-1732, doi:10.1007/s00134-006-0349-5 (2006).

[8] Malbrain, M. L. N. G., De laet, I. & Cheatham, M. CONSENSUS CONFERENCE DEFINITIONS AND RECOMMENDATIONS ON INTRA-ABDOMINAL HYPERTENSION (IAH) AND THE ABDOMINAL COMPARTMENT SYNDROME (ACS) - THE LONG ROAD TO THE FINAL PUBLICATIONS, HOW DID WE GET THERE? Acta Clinica Belgica 62, 44-59, doi:10.1179/acb.2007.62.s1.007 (2007).

[9] Malbrain, M. L. Different techniques to measure intra-abdominal pressure (IAP): time for a critical re-appraisal.

[10] Cheatham, M. L. Abdominal Compartment Syndrome: pathophysiology and definitions. Scandinavian Journal of Trauma, Resuscitation and Emergency Medicine 17, 10, doi:10.1186/1757-7241-17-10 (2009).

[11] Cheatham, M. L., White Mw Fau - Sagraves, S. G., Sagraves Sg Fau - Johnson, J. L., Johnson Jl Fau - Block, E. F. & Block, E. F. Abdominal perfusion pressure: a superior parameter in the assessment of intra-abdominal hypertension.

[12] Deeren, D. H., Dits H Fau - Malbrain, M. L. N. G. & Malbrain, M. L. Correlation between intra-abdominal and intracranial pressure in nontraumatic brain injury.

[13] Pickhardt, P. J., Shimony Js Fau - Heiken, J. P., Heiken Jp Fau - Buchman, T. G., Buchman Tg Fau - Fisher, A. J. & Fisher, A. J. The abdominal compartment syndrome: CT findings.

[14] Bouveresse, S. et al. Abdominal compartment syndrome and intra-abdominal hypertension in critically ill patients: diagnostic value of computed tomography.

[15] Patel, A., Lall Cg Fau - Jennings, S. G., Jennings Sg Fau - Sandrasegaran,

K. & Sandrasegaran, K. Abdominal compartment syndrome.

[16] Cheatham, M. L. & Safcsak, K. Intraabdominal pressure: a revised method for measurement.

[17] Davis, P. J., Koottayi S Fau - Taylor, A., Taylor A Fau - Butt, W. W. & Butt, W. W. Comparison of indirect methods of measuring intra-abdominal pressure in children.

[18] De Potter, T. J., Dits H Fau - Malbrain, M. L. N. G. & Malbrain, M. L. Intra- and interobserver variability during in vitro validation of two novel methods for intra-abdominal pressure monitoring.

[19] Gudmundsson, F. F., Viste A Fau - Gislason, H., Gislason H Fau - Svanes, K. & Svanes, K. Comparison of different methods for measuring intra-abdominal pressure.

[20] Balogh, Z., Jones F Fau - D'Amours, S., D'Amours S Fau - Parr, M., Parr M Fau - Sugrue, M. & Sugrue, M. Continuous intra-abdominal pressure measurement technique.

[21] Schachtrupp, A. et al. Evaluation of a modified piezoresistive technique and a water-capsule technique for direct and continuous measurement of intra-abdominal pressure in a porcine model.

[22] Schachtrupp, A. et al. Evaluation of two novel methods for the direct and continuous measurement of the intra-abdominal pressure in a porcine model.

[23] De Waele, J., Pletinckx P Fau - Blot, S., Blot S Fau - Hoste, E. & Hoste, E. Saline volume in transvesical intra-abdominal pressure measurement: enough is enough.

[24] De Waele Jj Fau - Billiet, E. A. I., Billiet Ea Fau - Hoste, E., Hoste E Fau - Blot, S. I., Blot Si Fau - Colardyn, F. A. & Colardyn, F. A. Fluid vs. air for semicontinuous intra-abdominal pressure measurements using a compliance catheter.

[25] Bitar, Z. A.-O. et al. The use of point-of-care ultrasound to guide clinical management in intra-abdominal hypertension. LID - 10.1007/s40477-020-00546-8 [doi].

[26] Tyson, N. & Efthymiou, C. Predictive risk factors for intra-abdominal hypertension after cardiac surgery. LID - ivaa336 [pii] LID - 10.1093/icvts/ivaa336 [doi].

[27] van Brunschot, S. et al. Abdominal compartment syndrome in acute pancreatitis: a systematic review.

[28] Singh, B. et al. Hypertriglyceridemia induced pancreatitis complicated by compartment syndrome and managed by surgical decompression and plasmapheresis.

[29] Muresan, M. et al. How much does decompressive laparotomy reduce the mortality rate in primary abdominal compartment syndrome?: A single-center prospective study on 66 patients.

[30] Schwenter, A., Schuepfer, G., Beck, M. & Mauch, J. Abdominal compartment syndrome after hip arthroscopy.

[31] Sharma, A., Sachdev H Fau - Gomillion, M. & Gomillion, M. Abdominal compartment syndrome during hip arthroscopy.

[32] Shakuo, T., Bito, K., Yasuda, S. & Asagi, C. Abdominal compartment syndrome during hip arthroscopy for an acetabular fracture: a case report.

[33] Ciemniewska-Gorzela, K., Piontek T Fau - Szulc, A. & Szulc, A. Abdominal compartment syndrome--the prevention and treatment of possible lethal complications following hip arthroscopy: a case report.

[34] Wise R Fau - Jacobs, J. et al. Incidence and prognosis of intra-abdominal hypertension and abdominal compartment syndrome in severely burned patients: Pilot study and review of the literature.

[35] Cheatham, M. L. & Safcsak, K. Percutaneous Catheter Decompression in the Treatment of Elevated Intraabdominal Pressure. CHEST 140, 1428-1435, doi:10.1378/chest.10-2789 (2011).

[36] Patel, A., Davis, C. & Davis, T. Percutaneous catheter drainage of secondary abdominal compartment syndrome: A case report.

[37] Dubose, J. J. et al. Open abdominal management after damage-control laparotomy for trauma: a prospective observational American Association for the Surgery of Trauma multicenter study.

[38] Hsu, Y.-P. et al. Analysis for Patient Survival after Open Abdomen for Torso Trauma and the Impact of Achieving Primary Fascial Closure: A Single-Center Experience. Sci Rep 8, 6213 (2018). <http://europepmc.org/abstract/MED/29670226

[39] Kreis, B. E., de Mol van Otterloo Aj Fau - Kreis, R. W. & Kreis, R. W. Open abdomen management: a review of its history and a proposed management algorithm.

[40] Cannon, J. W. et al. Damage control resuscitation in patients with severe traumatic hemorrhage: A practice management guideline from the Eastern Association for the Surgery of Trauma.

[41] Demetriades, D. & Salim, A. Management of the open abdomen.

[42] Sugrue, M. Abdominal compartment syndrome and the open abdomen: any unresolved issues?

Section 4

Diagnosis of Compartment Syndrome

Chapter 5

Non-Invasive Diagnostics in Acute Compartment Syndrome

Richard Martin Sellei, Philipp Kobbe and Frank Hildebrand

Abstract

Diagnosis of acute compartment syndrome (ACS) of the extremities is based on clinical signs with or without complementary measurement of muscle compartmental pressure. However, in cases of imminent compartment syndrome, unconscious patients or children the appropriate diagnose remains challenging. Despite all efforts to improve technical devices to objectify the signs by measurements of numerous parameters, needle compartment pressure measurement is to date accepted as the gold standard to facilitate decision making. But its invasiveness, the controversy about pressure thresholds and its potentially limited validity due to a single measurement support the need for further developments to diagnose ACS. Numerous technical improvements have been published and revealed promising new applications for non-invasive diagnostics. Since the pathology of an ACS is well characterized two approaches of measurements are described: to detect either increasing compartmental pressure or decreasing perfusion pressure. In the following, currently known investigations are reviewed and related to their pathophysiological principals, modes of clinical application, value and reliability.

Keywords: diagnostics, non-invasive, acute compartment syndrome, technical approaches

1. Introduction

Acute compartment syndrome (ACS) is characterized by an increasing intracompartmental pressure (ICP) provoked by intrinsic or extrinsic reasons [1, 2]. The consecutive muscle swelling due to a decreased perfusion pressure results in an impaired microcirculation and an additional increase of ICP [3]. The rise in venous pressure and cellular hypoxia causes further tissue oedema and swelling within the compartment finally concluding in the vicious circle of ACS [1, 4]. Numerous cases of different causes and heterogenous clinical appearances of ACS are presented in the literature. Differences in the velocity and severity of ACS development lead to a substantial heterogeneity of clinical findings. The initial clinical suspicion and awareness about a possible ACS by the physician itself is one of the most important issues not to miss the diagnose. The history and clinical findings of the affected patient alone resulted in a low positive predictive value. However, the negative predictive value to exclude an ACS by the clinician is as high as 98% [5]. The prompt diagnosis of the ACS is crucial to obviate the potential devastating clinical results after an overlooked or delayed recognition of an ACS. Hence, there is a reasonable need for complementary technical applications to facilitate and to objectify the presented condition of the muscle compartment. This uncertainty in diagnostics finally results in a high probability of over diagnose ACS following unnecessary fasciotomies.

2. Diagnostics and clinical investigations in ACS

By reason of continued controversy regarding the value and interpretation of compartmental pressure monitoring numerous scientific approaches have published over the last three decades. To date, none of the innovative techniques persuaded the clinician to replace invasive compartmental pressure monitoring by a new instrument or application. This certainty allows to conclude, that further developments of basic investigations are needed to assess either the increasing pressure or the decreasing perfusion pressure. The desired innovation of an additional technical investigation should provide specific requirements:

- Non-invasiveness
- Simplicity and possible repetitive/continuous application
- Clear threshold for the need of surgical intervention
- High inter- and intra-observer reliability
- Low cost and easily available application

Regarding the mentioned requirements different approaches are conceivable to achieve the improvements in clinical investigations (**Figure 1**).

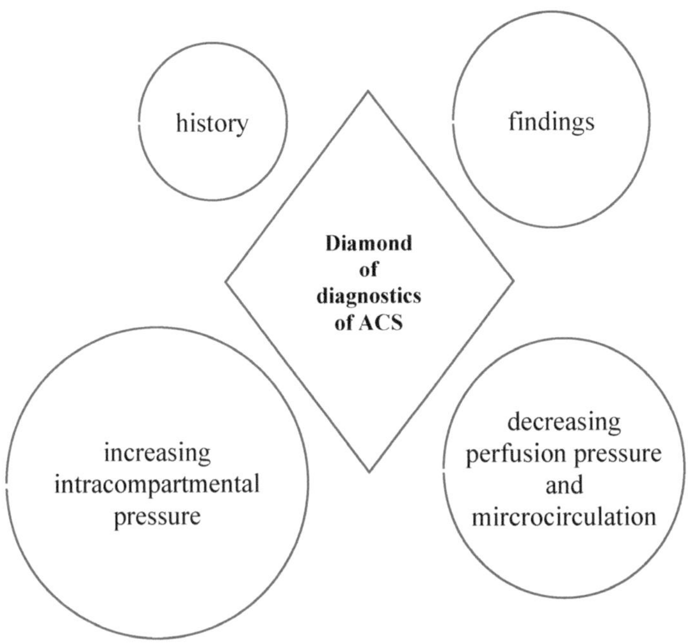

Figure 1.
The suspicion of an ACS allows to pursue the assumed diagnosis. The history of injury, the clinical findings and objectified diagnostics lead to the diagnosis or disclosure of an ACS. Decreased perfusion pressure provokes a disturbed microcirculation and results in increasing intra-compartmental pressure by a proceeding oedema. These four pathophysiological columns create the basic principles of diagnostics: The diamond of diagnostics of ACS.

3. Non-invasive diagnostics in acute compartment syndrome

3.1 Clinical findings

The clinical findings of the clinician are caused by one of the two fundamental pathophysiological mechanisms such as decreasing perfusion pressure with compromised microcirculation and/or increased intra-compartmental pressure. These two major mechanisms aggravate each other and lead to the clinical red flag signs summarized by the seven P's (pressure, pain out of proportion, pain with passive stretching, paresthesia, paresis, pink skin color, pulses present) [6]. As a result of a major uncertainty to indicate fasciotomy by clinical assessment only, the technical efforts in innovations concentrate on changes of the above mentioned parameters.

3.2 How can we objectify our findings non-invasively?

Many excellent approaches have been published over the last decades to objectify the parameters in order to exclude ACS or to substantiate imminent such as acute compartment syndrome. All of them can be categorized by terms of the pathology and parameter which is measured. The non-invasive approaches to diagnose ACS can be discriminated by the detection of a decreased perfusion pressure and reduced microcirculation or the increased pressure within the muscle compartment (**Table 1**).

Non-invasive diagnostics and measurements of ACS pathophysiology

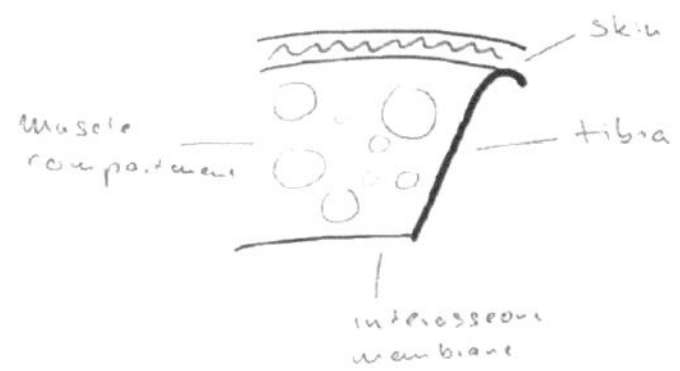

	Decreasing perfusion pressure		Increasing compartmental pressure
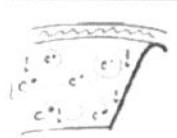	Infrared imaging	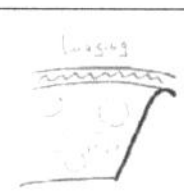	Imaging
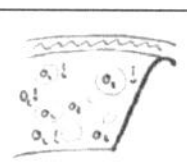	Pulse oximetry	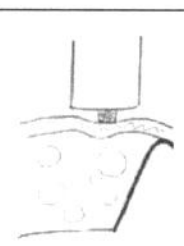	Tissue hardness measurement
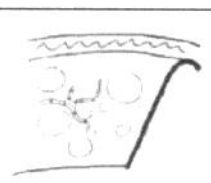	Laser doppler flowmetry (LDF)	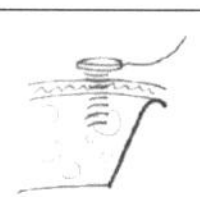	Pulsed phase locked loop ultrasound (PPLL)
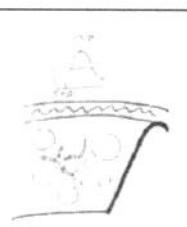	Contrast enhanced ultrasound (CEUS)	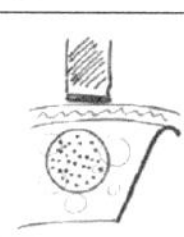	Shear wave elastography (SWE)
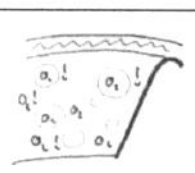	Near-infrared spectroscopy (NIRS)	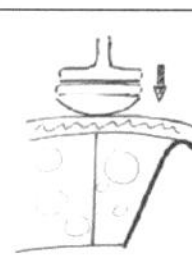	Pressure related ultrasound (PRUS)

Table 1.
Non-invasive approaches of diagnostics to identify and to objectify an acute compartment syndrome.

4. Noninvasive measurement of surrogates of decreased perfusion pressure

4.1 Infrared imaging

Infrared imaging to measure the surface temperature was used to detect ACS of the affected lower leg by comparison with the uninjured limb. The aim of this application was to use a portable and non-invasive technology, for detecting ACS in patients with multiple trauma [7]. The hypothesized reduction in surface temperature has been proven in a clinical study. The authors used an index of temperature measurements of the proximal vs. distal limb (thigh-foot-index) and showed a significant difference in patients developing ACS in 167 cases. They concluded that infrared imaging may support early detection of ACS in trauma patients based on correlation between a decreasing perfusion pressure and an increased difference of the temperature index. However, thresholds of the index are difficult to define, especially in trauma patients.

4.2 Pulse oximetry

Pulse oximetry was examined to detect the decreasing perfusion pressure in case of ACS as it has been advocated as a simple non-invasive investigation of vascular compromise nearly thirty years ago [8]. Whilst a significant decrease of oxygen saturation was detected, the sensitivity of 40% was low. Therefore, this application was conceded [9].

4.3 Pulsed doppler ultrasound

Mc Loughlin et al. hypothesized that a diastolic retrograde arterial flow (DRAF) may represent an early sign of ACS. They therefore mimicked a compartment syndrome by using a cuff inducing external compression of the forearm with increasing pressure in two patients. The authors showed a strong correlation of DRAF (%) with the degree of external pressure applied and concluded that this technique may represent a useful tool in detection and evaluation of ACS [9]. To our knowledge no further work was published pursuing this application.

4.4 Laser doppler flowmetry

Abraham et al. investigated the direct measurement of muscle blood flow with laser doppler flowmetry (LDF) compared with the intracompartmental pressure measurement in patients with chronic compartment syndrome (CCS) [10]. In the CCS group a delayed hyperaemic peak in muscle blood flow was detected. They concluded that LDF should be investigated further as a technique for diagnosis of CCS. In the literature, no evaluation of LDF in ACS was found.

4.5 Contrast enhanced ultrasound (CEUS)

Geis et al. used contrast enhancement in ultrasound to detect the compromised perfusion pressure and to monitor changes of microcirculation in ACS. In a clinical study, eight patients with ACS underwent a B-mode ultrasound examination using a multifrequence probe. An intravenous bolus injection of a contrast agent resulted in a colored visualization of microperfusion. A time-intensity-curve was analyzed retrospectively and quantified by a software. Parameters as time-to arrival (TTA), peak of signal intensity (%), time-to peak (TTP), the regional blood volume (RBV), the regional blood flow (RBF), and the mean-transit-time (MTT) were calculated and resulted in significant differences in case of ACS [11]. The authors concluded that CEUS may be capable of differing between ACS and an imminent compartment syndrome. These results were supported by a volunteer study with a simulated decrease of perfusion pressure by torniquet of the thigh [12]. However, the bolus application of a contrast agent and its possible undesirable effects, particularly in patients with pre-existing cardio-vascular illness, refuses further clinical application of this technology.

4.6 Near-infrared spectroscopy (NIRS)

The invasive measurement of the oxygen partial pressure has been examined in animal models [13] and in clinical studies [14]. These investigations demonstrated a correlation of decreasing local muscle tissue oxygenation and increasing pressure due to ACS. The sensitivity and specificity of the partial pressure oxygenation of less than 30 mmHg as a threshold in an animal model showed excellent results [15] and have been confirmed in a non-invasive technique of oxygen saturation measurement by near-infrared spectroscopy (NIRS) [16]. This approach assessed the level of oxygenated muscle hemoglobin and muscle myoglobin. With the decreased blood flow after trauma-induced ACS, a reduction in local oxygen saturation as well as oxygen tension was detected [17]. In animal models, NIRS showed a clear correlation between decreased tissue oxygenation and reduced muscle perfusion pressure [18]. In further clinical studies using NIRS, the strength of non-invasive techniques for monitoring of affected limbs was emphasized [19, 20].

However, the reliability of NIRS measurements as a single parameter in monitoring ACS showed poor values [21]. The main limitations in this approach are constrained depth of penetration (30-40 mm), variables affecting penetration and reflection of radiated infrared light signal (e.g. melanin), the lack of appropriate threshold for ACS indicating fasciotomy and the effect of hypotension and hypoxia in trauma patients on the measurement. However, with further technical developments NIRS has the potential to be used in monitoring trauma patients with imminent compartment syndrome or even be able to indicate the need for surgical intervention.

4.7 Dynamic phosphorous-31 magnetic resonance spectroscopy

Recently Otha et al. utilized dynamic phosphorous-31 magnetic resonance spectroscopy (^{31}P-MRS) for visualization of metabolic changes as surrogate of muscle ischemia in an animal model [22]. ^{31}P-MRS is able to dynamically monitor the rate of inorganic phosphate (Pi) depletion and synthesis, phosphocreatine (PCr), intracellular pH and mitochondrial oxidative capacity. They demonstrated a significant decrease of the PCr/(Pi+PCr) ratio after inducing ischemia in an ACS model with rats. The intracellular and arterial pH index also decreased over time significantly. The authors concluded, that this noninvasive imaging approach rapidly detects metabolic changes in the muscle compartment and may represent a non-invasive method for determining early damage in ACS in the future.

4.8 Phonomyography

Martinez et al. used acoustic myography (Phonomyography) to measure the degree of muscle ischemia in an animal model [23]. After 30 minutes of simulated ischemia, the signal from the calf musculature provoked by stimulation of the sciatic nerve in the thigh, decreased significantly at 55%. At 120 minutes of ischemia, the signal dropped at 68%. In conclusion, the authors recognized phonomyography as a non-invasive method for continuous monitoring of patients with ACS.

5. Noninvasive measurement of surrogates of increased intra-compartmental pressure

5.1 Imaging

The imaging of muscle compartments developing an ACS was insufficient to detect early morphological changes. B-mode ultrasound imaging [24] as well as MRI imaging [25] was described as potential methods to detect severe pathologies (e.g. muscle swelling or necrosis). However, imaging alone does not reliably detect pathological changes in an early stage of an ACS. In a clinical study, Gershuni et al. identified a correlation between enhanced pressure and increasing volume of the tibial anterior compartment after exercise by B-mode ultrasound in the cross-section view [26]. Rajasekaran et al. presented a significant increase in muscle compartment thickness in patients with chronic exertional compartment syndrome compared with control subjects after exertion using ultrasound [27]. Wang et al. measured the thickness of the anterior compartment in twenty acute trauma cases. The thickness and the ICP were significantly increased compared to the uninjured lower limb, but the increase in ICP did not show a significant correlation with the change in thickness of the injured lower leg [28].

Beside the thickness of the compartment in a feasibility study, the ultrasound-guided angle measurement as a surrogate of increased pressure was investigated in a human cadaver model of ACS. The authors measured the tibia-fascia angle (TFA) between the anterolateral cortex of the tibia and the tangent to the curving anterior compartment fascia with its origin at the tibial attachment. Measurements in forty specimens resulted in a mean TFA of 61.0° (± 12°) at 10 mmHg. Each increase in pressure by 3.9 mmHg was associated with an increase of TFA by one degree. The inter-observer reliability was good (ICC 0.77). The authors concluded that the increasing ICP of the anterior tibial compartment can be estimated well by ultrasound-based TFA measurement post mortem. However, the authors also stated that the findings are too preliminary to be used in clinical practice [29].

5.2 Tissue hardness measurement

Over the last three decades non-invasive diagnostic principles have been introduced and enhanced. Several authors showed promising results when investigating the soft-tissue elasticity. In a study of 75 cases of suspected ACS, a noninvasive hardness measuring device was included. Upper and lower extremities were tested. ICP pressure values and hardness ratios were compared to one another as continuous variables. Due to the low specificity of the noninvasive measurement of hardness compared to the invasive pressure measurement, the authors concluded that the use of the hardness monitor has no potential to determine the diagnosis of compartment syndrome [30]. In a feasibility study of healthy volunteers and patients with chronic myofascial neck pain syndrome a soft tissue stiffness meter was evaluated to measure the soft tissue stiffness (STS) in the form of the instantaneous force (N) by which the tissue resists the constant deformation produced by a cylindrical intender. The resulting data of a hand-held computerized soft tissue stiffness meter (STSM) in index muscles (e.g. m. trapezius and m. levator scapulae muscle) resulted in a linear, positive relationship between the indenter force (N) and the dynamic compressive modulus (MPa) of elastomer stiffness. The authors concluded that STSM assessment can evaluate the tissue stiffness quantitatively and yield reproducible data [31]. Steinberg et al. first introduced in 1994 a hardness meter to determine the quantitative muscle compartment hardness in six dogs and three anatomical specimen limbs simulation ACS by plasma injection into the index compartment. In six patients with suspected ACS the quantitative muscle hardness also was measured and compared with the uninjured limb. The authors showed a close correlation between the direct measurement of ICP with the wick catheter and quantitative hardness in compartment syndrome models in dog and anatomic specimen limbs, and in patients suspected of having compartment syndromes. They concluded, that the determination of surface hardness of limb muscle compartments, which appears accurate and reproducible, offers the advantages of being noninvasive and well suited for longer-term assessments of ICP [32]. Further development of this device showed promising results in a study of eighteen volunteers simulating an increased ICP in a torniquet model. The results showed a statistically significant strong linear relationship between the ICP and the quantitative hardness measurement. Again, the authors concluded that quantitative hardness measurements may accurately predict ICP for most patients. This technique may greatly enhance the medical community's ability to diagnose compartment syndrome with a noninvasive means [33].

The use of quantitative muscle compartment hardness measurement finally was examined in a large cohort of 205 patients with ACS by two independent observers resulting in a strong overall correlation of hardness measurement and ICP. The authors concluded that the quantitative hardness is potentially useful for the monitoring of IMP elevation in compartment syndrome [34]. These studies confirm that the presented approach of objectifying the clinical findings by the observer may have the potential for the future to monitor, predict and determine the need for fasciotomy in better modes than today. However, there is still a need for a reliable tool assessing the soft-tissue swelling to objectify the clinical findings by further developments.

5.3 Pulsed phase locked loop (PPLL) ultrasound

A further approach to determine a parameter correlated with the decreased ICP is the portable technique of ultrasonic pulsed phase locked loop (PPLL) technology. With this method the myofascial displacement is detected after stimulation with an ultrasonic impulse. The difference in frequency of the transmitted ultrasonic impulse and the detected reflection is measured. Linear displacements of the myofascial layer that result from the arterial pulse can be detected. Lynch et al. transferred this technology to determine decreasing myofascial displacements in ACS with increasing ICP [35]. In several studies they showed a strong non-linear correlation between the PPLL measurements and the direct ICP determination in ex-vivo and animal models [35, 36]. This correlation with increasing ICP also was proven in a study with healthy volunteers [37] and patients with ACS [38]. The demonstrated results showed remarkable sensitivity of 75% and specificity of 75%. Because of the non-linear correlation with the ICP and the arterial pulse amplitude interpretation concerns were raised regarding the PPLL technology especially in trauma patients with hypotension. Further studies may deliver more data that support this technique in noninvasive monitoring of ACS.

5.4 Elastography

Ultrasound elastography was introduced in the early 1990s [39, 40]. It allows to differentiate the mechanical properties of tissue by qualitative visual or quantitative measurements [41]. Over the last three decades, this technique evolved into a tool for real-time imaging of the distribution of tissue strain in relation to its elastic modulus. The most common technique of stress application is the strain (compression, real-time) ultrasound elastography [42]. Low-frequency compression on the soft tissue (e.g. breast, abdominal organs, muscle) is usually applied manually with a hand-held B-mode transducer. The resulting axial tissue displacement or strain provokes different echo sets before and after compression, which are visualized by different colors. Thus, ultrasound elastography provides information on relative tissue stiffness compared with the adjacent and surrounding tissue within the image section. There is limited date available on the use of real-time elastography for skeletal muscle [43, 44]. Niitsu et al. described in a feasibility study in healthy volunteers the potential measurement of muscle hardness calculating the "strain ratio" by the relative elasticity of the biceps muscle compared to that of the reference before and after exercise [43]. These results were supported by a study in seven volunteers after muscle exercise [45]. Toyoshima et al. recently demonstrated the feasibility of soft tissue elasticity measurement based on ultrasound shear wave elastography (SWE). The elastic modulus of tissue was estimated from shear wave speed (SWS; m/sec) induced by acoustic radiation force of a focused ultrasound beam. In an ex-vivo animal model with turkey hind limbs increasing ICP was simulated in the anterior-lateral and anterior-deep compartment. A strong correlation was observed between the increasing ICP and increasing SWS measurements. The authors concluded, that the ICP can be accurately measured by using ultrasound shear wave elastography [46]. However, further clinical studies are needed to prove the concept of SWE in patients with ACS.

5.5 Pressure related ultrasound (PRUS)

The use of B-mode ultrasound combined with a pressure sensor can be used to determine the muscle hardness. Muraki et al. investigated whether a combination of the thickness and hardness of muscles without muscle tension is feasible to estimate muscle strength of the anterior thigh during knee extension in adult volunteers. A compression ratio (%) of the muscle thickness before and after compression (10 N) using an internal coiled spring resulted in a significant positive correlation with the strength [47].

The probe pressure-related use of B-mode ultrasound to estimate compartment pressure was first described in a basic in-vitro model [48]. In this context, the ratio (%) between the compartment depth in a condition without compression compared to a state with a defined pressure by the ultrasound probe (100 mmHg) was calculated. The authors demonstrated a strong non-linear correlation between a decreasing compression depth and an increasing ICP with a Pearson correlation coefficient of $r^2 = 0.960$. The results in this feasibility study were confirmed in a cadaver study. The authors concluded that pressure-related ultrasound (PRUS) could be a reliable tool to determine the correlation between the measured compartmental displacement and the increasing ICP [49]. Bloch et al. tested this experimental setup of compression sonography in an animal model in six domestic pig legs. Increasing ICP in the anterior tibial compartment was simulated in 5 mmHg steps. The elasticity ratio (%) significantly differed from the baseline measurement compared with the simulated pressure of 30 and 40 mmHg. A compression ratio less than 12.9% had a sensitivity of 94.4% and a specificity of 89% to proper diagnose ACS. The authors concluded, that compression sonography might offer a non-invasive technique help in cases of uncertain ACS [50]. In a prospective study in six patients with verified ACS the muscle compartment elasticity of the injured lower limb was compared with the uninjured limb. This comparison resulted in a significant difference of the compression ratio (%) using PRUS [51]. The uninjured anterior tibial compartment resulted in a ratio of 17.95% (SD +/− 5), whereas the injured limbs showed ratios of 5,14% (+/− 2) and thereby was significantly different. A ratio less than 10.5% had a sensitivity of 95.8% and a specificity of 87.5% to properly diagnose ACS. Therewith the results of the previously described animal model were confirmed. Marmor et al. used PRUS to determine the pressure at the condition of flattening the concave myofascial layer. In this cadaver study significant differences for the compartment fascia flattening pressure (CFFP) between the control and the simulated ACS group were demonstrated. The authors suggested that there is a potential for the clinical use of this modality in the future [52]. These results recently have been confirmed in a prospective clinical study in fifty-two patients with tibial fractures. The CFFP in the injured limbs resulted in a significant difference compared with the uninjured lower leg with good to excellent inter- and intra-observer agreements [53]. The inter- and intra-observer reliability of PRUS was recently investigated in a blinded in-vitro model in twelve volunteers [54]. This study confirmed a very high reproducibility of measurements (ICC_{inter} of 0,986 and ICC_{intra} of 0,985). Further technical improvements and clinical studies are required to implement this application in clinical scenario.

6. Conclusion

To date, the diagnosis of ACS is based on the suspicion in history of the patient, the clinical findings and in cases of uncertainty supported by invasive ICP measurements. There is an unambiguous need for further technical approaches to objectify ether the decreasing perfusion pressure and microcirculation or the increasing intra-compartmental pressure within the myofascial layer to measure the condition of suspected ACS. In the literature, numerous publications demonstrate the difficulty of a clear and precise determination of the condition within the suspected muscle compartment. Subsequently, sometimes unnecessary or delayed fasciotomies are inevitably provoked. Thus, the requirements of an ideal approach to objectify a suspected ACS is easy to determine. A non-invasive, reliable, low-cost and easy monitoring with defined threshold to determine fasciotomy is needed.

The above described technical innovations and applications aspire to fulfill these requirements. The measurement of the decreasing perfusion pressure seems to be more sensitive to detect early changes in the diamond concept of ACS diagnostics. In respect of the complex and dynamic changes of the muscle compartment condition the combination of different approaches may solve the mentioned requirements in the future.

At this point in time, none of these modalities have come into widespread use and the gold standard currently remains clinical examination and compartment pressure monitoring and if in doubt, it would be better to decompress an ACS to save the limb. Further developments and refinements are needed in the present non-invasive methods to make them more robust in contributing to the diagnosis of ACS.

Author details

Richard Martin Sellei[1,2*], Philipp Kobbe[2] and Frank Hildebrand[2]

1 Department of Orthopaedic Trauma, Sana Klinikum Offenbach, Offenbach am Main, Germany

2 Department of Orthopaedic Trauma and Reconstructive Surgery, University of Aachen Medical Center, Aachen, Germany

*Address all correspondence to: richard.sellei@sana.de

References

[1] Schmid AH. Acute compartment syndrome. Injury. 2017; 48:S22-S25.

[2] Garner MR, Taylor SA, Gausden E, Lyden JP. Compartment syndrome: Diagnosis, management, and unique concerns in the twenty-first century. HSS J. 2014; 10:143-152.

[3] Hansen EN, Manzano G, Kandemir U, Mok JM. Comparison of tissue oxygenation and compartment pressure following tibia fracture. Injury. 2013; 44:1076-1080.

[4] Rorabeck CH, Clarke KM. The pathophysiology of anterior tibial compartment syndrome: An experimental investigation. J Trauma. 1978; 18:299-304.

[5] Ulmer T. The clinical diagnosis of compartment syndrome of the lower leg: Are clinical finding predictive of the disorder? J Orthop Trauma. 2002; 16: 572-577.

[6] Von Keudell AG, Weaver MJ, Appleton PT, Bae DS, Dyer GSM, Heng M, Jupiter JB Vrahas MS. Diagnosis and treatment of acute extremity compartment syndrome. Lancet. 2015; 386:1299-1310

[7] Katz LM, Nauriyal V, Nagaraj S, Finsch A, Pearlstein K, Szymanowski A, Sproule C, Rich PB, Guenther BD, Pearlstein RD. Infrared imaging of trauma patients for detection of acute compartment syndrome of the lag. Crit Care Med. 2008; 36:1756-1761

[8] Mars M, Hadley GP. Failure of pulse oximetry in the assessment of raised limb intracompartmental pressure. Injury. 1994; 25:379-381

[9] Mac Loughlin S, Ma Loughlin MJ, Mateu F. Pulsed Doppler in simulated compartment syndrome: A pilot study to record hemodynamic compromise. Ochsner J. 2013; 13:500-506

[10] Abraham P, Leftheriotis G, Saumet JL. Laser Doppler Flowmetry in diagnosis of chronic compartment syndrome. J Bone Joint Surg. 1998; 80-B: 365-369

[11] Geis S, Gehnert S, Lamby P, Zellner J, Pfeifer C, Prantl L, Jung EM. Contrast enhanced ultrasound (CEUS) and time intensity curve (TIC) analysis in compartment syndrome: First results. Clin Hemorheol Microcirc. 2012; 50:1-11

[12] Sellei RM, Waehling A, Weber CD, Jeromin S, Zimmermann F, McCann PA, Hildebrand F, Pape HC. Contrast enhanced ultrasound (CEUS) reliably detects critical perfusion changes in compartmental muscle: A model in healthy volunteers. Eur J Trauma Emerg Surg. 2014; 40:535-539

[13] Weick JW, Kang H, Lee L, Kuether J, Liu X, Hansen EN, Kandemir U, Rollins, Mok JM. Direct measurement of tissue oxygenation as a method of diagnosis of acute compartment syndrome. J Orthop Trauma. 2016; 30: 585-591

[14] Hansen EN, Manzano G, Kandemir U, Mok JM. Comparison of tissue oxygenation and compartment pressure following tibia fracture. Injury. 2013; 44: 1076-1080

[15] Doro CJ, Sitzman TJ, O'Toole RV. Can intramuscular glucose levels diagnose compartment syndrome? J Trauma Acute Care Surg. 2014; 76: 474-478

[16] Reisman WM, Shuler MS, Roskosky M, Kinsey TL, Freedman BA. Use of near-infrared spectroscopy to detect sustained hyperaemia following lower extremity trauma. Mil Med. 2016; 181:111-115

[17] Lee SH, Padilla M, Lynch JE, Hargens AR. Noninvasive measurement

of pressure of detecting compartment syndromes. J Orthop Rheumatol. 2013; 1:5

[18] Budsberg SC, Shuler MS, Hansen M, Uhl E, Freedman BA. Comparison of NIRS, serum biomarkers, and muscle damage in a porcine balloon compression model of acute compartment syndrome. J Trauma Acute Care Surg. 2016; 81:876-881

[19] Shuler MS, Roskosky M, Kinsey T, Glaser D, Reisman W, Ogburn C, Yeoman C, Wanderman NR, Freedman B. Continual near-infrared spectroscopy monitoring in the injured lower limb and acute compartment syndrome. B Joint J. 2018; 100-B:181-797

[20] Tobias JD, Hoernschemeyer DG. Near-infrared spectroscopy identifies compartment syndrome in an infant. J Paediatric Orthop. 2007; 27:311-313

[21] Schmidt A, Bossee M, O'Toole R, Obremsky W, Zipunnikov V, Dunrui D, Rey K, MacKenzie E. Continous near-infrared spectroscopy monitoring in the injured lower limb and compartment syndrome. Bone Joint J. 2018; 100-B: 787-797

[22] Ohta H, Van Vo NM, Hata J, Terawaki K, Shirakawa T, Okano HJ. Utilizing dynamic phosphorous-31 magnetic resonance spectroscopy for early detection of acute compartment syndrome: A pilot study on rats. Diagnostics. 2021; 11:586-601

[23] Martinez AP, Moser TP, Saran N, Paquet M, Hemmerling T, Berry GK. Phonomyography as a non-invasive continuous monitoring technique for muscle ischemia in an experimental model of acute compartment syndrome. Injury. 2017; 48: 2411-2416

[24] Jerosch J, Geske B, Sons HU, Winkelmann W. The value of sonography in assessing intracompartmental pressure in the anterior tibial compartment. Ultraschall Med. 1989; 10:206-210

[25] Correa DG, Costa FM, Mendonca S, Severo A, Canella C. Magnetic Resonance Imaging Alterations in Acute Compartment Syndrome. J Foot Ankle Surg. 2021; ahead of print; doi: 10.1053/j.jfas.2019.10.006

[26] Gershuni DH, Gosink BB, Hargens AR, Gould RN, Forsythe JR, Mubarak SJ. Ultrasound evaluation of the anterior musculofascial compartment of the leg following exercise. Clin Orthop Rel Res. 1982; 167: 185–190

[27] Rajasekaran S, Beavis C, Aly AR, Leswick D. The utility of ultrasound in detecting anterior compartment thickness changes in chronic exertional compartment syndrome: A pilot study. Clin J Sport Med. 2013; 23:305–311

[28] Wang SH, Lin KY, Yang JJ, Chang JH, Huang GS, Lin LC. The thickness of the anterior compartment does not indicate compartment syndrome in acutely traumatized legs? Injury. 2014; 45:578-582

[29] Muehlbacher J, Pauzenberger R, Asenbaum U, Gauster T, Kapral S, Herkner H, Duma A. Feasibility of ultrasound measurement in a human model of acute compartment syndrome. World J Emerg Surg. 2019; 14:4; doi: 10.1186/s13017-019-0222-9

[30] Dickson KF, Sullivan MJ, Steinberg B. Noninvasive measurement of compartment syndrome. Orthopedics. 2003; 26:1215–1218

[31] Arokoski JPA, Surakka J, Ojala T, Arokoski JP, Surakka J, Ojala T, et al. Feasibility of the use of a novel soft tissue stiffness meter. Physiol Meas. 2005; 26:215–228

[32] Steinberg BD, Gelberman RH. Eva luation of limb compartment with suspected increased interstitial pressure.

A noninvasive method for determining quantitative hardness. Clin Orthop Relat Res. 1994; 300:248-53

[33] Steinberg BD. Evaluation of limb compartments with increased interstitial pressure. An improved noninvasive method for determining quantitative hardness. J Biomech. 2005; 38:1629–1635

[34] Steinberg B, Riel R, Armitage M, Berrey H. Quantitative muscle hardness as a noninvasive means for detecting pa tients at risk of compartment syndrome s. Physiol Meas. 2011 Apr;32(4):433-44. doi: 10.1088/0967-3334/32/4/005. Epub 2011 Mar 8.PMID: 21383493

[35] Lynch JE, Heyman JS, Hargens AR. Ultrasonic device for the noninvasive diagnosis of compartment syndrome. Physiol Meas. 2004; 25:N1-N9

[36] Lynch JE, Lynch JK, Cole SL, Carter JA, Hargens AR. Noninvasive monitoring of elevated intramuscular pressure in a model compartment syndrome via quantitative fascial motion. J Orthop Res. 2009; 27:489-494

[37] Lee SH, Padilla M, Lynch JE, Hargens AR. Noninvasive measurement of pressure for detecting compartment syndrome. J Orthop Rheumatol. 2013; 1:5

[38] Wiemann JM, Ueno T, Leek BT, Yost WT, Schwartz AK, Hargens AR. Noninvasive mesurements of intramuscular pressure using pulsed phase-locked loop ultrasound for detecting compartment syndromes: A preliminary report. J Orthop Trauma. 2006; 20:458-463

[39] Ophir J, Cespedes I, Ponnekanti H, Yazdi Y, Li X. Elastography: A quantitative method for imaging the elasticity of biological tissues. Ultrasound Imaging. 1991; 13:111–134.

[40] Lerner RM, Huang SR, Parker KJ. "Sonoelasticity" images derives from ultrasound signals in mechanically vibrated tissues. Ultrasound Med Biol. 1990; 16:231–239

[41] Garra BS. Imaging and estimation of tissue elasticity by ultrasound. Ultrasound. 2007; 23:255–268

[42] Park GY, Kwon DR. Application of real-time sonoelastography in musculoskeletal diseases related to physical medicine and rehabilitation. Am J Phys Med Rehabil. 2011; 90:875–886

[43] Niitsu M, Michizaki A, Endo A. Muscle hardness measurement by using ultrasound elastography: A feasibility study. Acta Radiol. 2011; 52:99–105

[44] Ariji Y, Katsumata A, Hiraiwa Y, Izumi M, Iida Y, Goto M, et al. Use of sonographic elastography of the masseter muscle for optimizing massage pressure: A preliminary study. J Oral Rehab. 2009; 36:627–635

[45] Yanagisawa O, Sakuma J, Kawakami Y, Suzuki K, Fukubayashi T. Effect of exercise-induced muscle damage on muscle hardness evaluated by ultrasound real-time tissue elastography. SpringerPlus. 2015; 2:308

[46] Toyoshima Y, Webb J, Gregory A, Fatemi M, Alizad A, Zhao C. Ultrasound shear wave elastography for measuring intracompartmental prerssure of compartment syndrome using a Turkey hind limb model. J Biomech. 2020; 98: 109427

[47] Muraki S, Fukumoto K, Fukuda O. Prediction of the muscle strength by the muscle thickness and hardness using ultrasound muscle hardness meter. SpringerPlus. 2013; 2:457-464

[48] Sellei RM, Hingmann SJ, Kobbe P, Weber CD, Grice JE, Zimmermann F, Jeromin S, Hildebrand F, Pape HC. Compartment elasticity measured by pressure-related ultrasound to determine patients "at risk" for compartment syndrome: An

experimental in vitro study. Patient Saf Surgery. 2015; 9:4-10

[49] Sellei RM, Hingmann SJ, Weber CD, Jeromin S, Zimmermann F, Turner J, Hildebrand F, Pape HC. Assessment of elevated compartment pressures by pressure-related ultrasound: A cadaveric model. Eur J Trauma Emerg Surg. 2015; 41:639.645

[50] Bloch A, Tomaschett C, Jakob SM, Schwinghammer A, Schmid T. Compression sonography for non-invasive measurement of lower leg compartment pressure in an animal model. Injury. 2018; 49:532-537

[51] Sellei RM, Wollnitz J, Reinhardt N, de la Fuente M, Radermacher K, Weber CD, Kobbe P, Hildebrand F. Non-invasive measurement of muscle compartment elasticity in lower limbs to determine acute compartment syndrome: Clinical results with pressure related ultrasound. Injury. 2020; 51: 301-306

[52] Marmor MT, Charlu J, Knox R, Curtis W, Hoogervorst P, Herfat S. Use of standard musculoskeletal ultrasound to determine the need for fasciotomy in an elevated muscle compartment pressure cadaver leg model. Injury. 2019; 50: 627-632

[53] Marmor MT, Barker JP, Matz J, Donohoe E, Herring MJ. A dual-sensor ultrasound based method for detecting elevated muscle compartment pressure: A prospective clinical pilot study. Injury. 2021; doi: 10.1016/j.injury. 2021.02.054.Online ahead of print

[54] Sellei RM, Warkotsch U, Kobbe P, Weber CD, Reinhard N, de la Fuente M, Radermacher K, Hildebrand F. Non-invasive and reliable assessment of compartment elasticity by pressure related ultrasound: An in-vitro study. Injury. 2020; doi: 10.1016/j.injury. 2020.10.069. Online ahead of print

Section 5

Compartment Syndrome in Special Situations

Chapter 6

Abdominal Compartment Syndrome among Medical Patients

Kejal Gandhi, Pahnwat Taweesedt, Munish Sharma, Dweep Barbhaya and Salim Surani

Abstract

Abdominal compartment syndrome and intra-abdominal hypertension (IAH) has been widely studied in surgical and trauma patients, even though the incidence of IAH in medical intensive care unit (MICU) remains high. Studies have shown that the time to decision making regarding diagnosis and management of IAH is twice in MICU compared to the corresponding surgical side. MICU patients often require large volume resuscitation such as in sepsis, hemorrhage, or an inflammatory condition such as acute pancreatitis, which increases the risk of development of IAH. It is often underdiagnosed and undertreated in MICU due to a lack of awareness of the consequences and mortality associated with it. Elevated intra-abdominal pressure has systemic effects causing atelectatic lungs, decreased cardiac output, and renal insufficiency. IAH, if not recognized early, can quickly progress to compartment syndrome causing multiorgan failure and death. Approach to ACS management between medical and surgical intensivists varies largely because of lack of experience with surgical decompression. This article provides an overview of definitions, incidence, pathophysiology, clinical presentation, diagnosis, and management of IAH and abdominal compartment syndrome in critically in medical patients.

Keywords: abdominal compartment syndrome, intra-abdominal hypertension, intra-abdominal pressure, medical intensive care unit, bladder pressure, multiorgan failure, decompression laparotomy

1. Introduction

A progressive increase in intra-abdominal pressure initially results in intra-abdominal hypertension and later, affects end-organ perfusion resulting in abdominal compartment syndrome. It is often under-diagnosed as the end-organ perfusion caused by intra-abdominal hypertension in this patient population can also be explained by their overall critical condition. Thus, clinicians must have a high suspicion for intra-abdominal hypertension to prevent it from progressing to compartment syndrome and death.

2. Definitions

2.1 Intra-abdominal pressure

The abdomen is a closed cavity with a steady state pressure within it. This pressure is called Intra-abdominal pressure (IAP). Intra-abdominal pressure depends on the abdominal wall compliance and volume of the organs within the abdominal cavity. Thus, it is affected by the conditions that decreases the compliance of the wall (burn eschars or third spacing) or by additional volume of organs (such as fecal matter, presence of ascites, or space-occupying lesions such as tumors) [1].

Normal IAP varies between 5–7 mmHg [2]. Body Mass Index positively affects IAP with pressure being high in pregnant and morbidly obese individuals. Similarly, recent abdominal surgery can also affect the IAP.

2.2 Abdominal perfusion pressure (APP)

Abdominal perfusion pressure (APP) is measured by subtraction of intra-abdominal pressure from the mean arterial pressure (MAP) [3].

$$APP = MAP - IAP \qquad (1)$$

With the increase in IAP, APP decreases, and thereby, causing decreased perfusion to the abdominal viscera. APP is a better maker than arterial pH, base deficit, arterial lactate and hourly urine output, as an endpoint for resuscitation.

2.3 Intra-abdominal hypertension (IAH)

The World Society of Abdominal Compartment Syndrome (WSACS) established the definition of IAH and ACS in 2004 [4].Intra-abdominal hypertension (IAH) is defined as intra-abdominal pressure (IAP) greater than or equal to 12 mmHg.

IAH is further graded based on the IAP as shown in **Table 1**.

IAH can also be divided as follows based on duration:

- Hyperacute IAH refers to the transient elevation of the intra-abdominal pressure lasting for seconds such as while laughing, sneezing, straining, coughing.
- Acute IAH refers to the sustained elevation of IAP over hours such as in intra-abdominal trauma or hemorrhage and has the potential to progress to ACS.
- Subacute IAH refers to the elevation of IAP over days and is mostly seen in the MICU patients receiving large volume resuscitation and also has potential to progress to ACS.

Grades	IAP
Grade I	12–15 mmHg
Grade II	16–20 mmHg
Grade III	21–25 mmHg
Grade IV	>25 mmHg

Table 1.
IAH classification based on IAP value [5].

- Chronic IAH refers to the elevation of IAP over months to years such as in patients with increased abdominal wall compliance (pregnant or morbidly obese). These patients are at high risk for development of ACS if they have superimposed acute or subacute IAH [6].

2.4 Filtration gradient (FG)

Oliguria is most often the first sign of IAH. FG is measured as glomerular filtration pressure (GFP) – PTP (proximal tubular pressure) and is a measure of pressure across the glomerulus.

$$GFP = MAP - IAP = APP \tag{2}$$

Since,

$$PTP = IAP \tag{3}$$

Therefore,

$$FG = GFP - PTP = (MAP - IAP) - IAP \tag{4}$$

Thus,

$$FG = MAP - 2xIAP \tag{5}$$

This equation shows that changes in IAP have a higher effect on renal function and urine production than changes in MAP [7].

2.5 Abdominal compartment syndrome (ACS)

Abdominal compartment syndrome (ACS) is defined as sustained IAP above 20 mmHg with evidence of end-organ dysfunction. ACS is further classified into primary, secondary, and recurrent based on the etiology and duration of end-organ failure.

Primary: ACS occurring due to etiology primarily within the abdominopelvic cavity is termed as primary; for example, abdominal trauma, pancreatitis, abdominal surgery, hemoperitoneum, liver transplantation. It frequently requires early surgical or interventional radiology intervention [8].

Secondary: ACS occurring due to extra-abdominal etiology; example: fluid resuscitation, sepsis, burns.

Recurrent: Development of ACS again after the early resolution of the previous either primary or secondary ACS. It can occur despite the presence of an open abdomen or after abdominal closure following the resolution of the first episode. It is associated with significant morbidity and mortality [9].

3. Incidence

Abdominal compartment syndrome has been studied widely in surgical and trauma patients. However, very few studies are available on the MICU patients. Many patients in MICU undergo large-volume resuscitation common conditions such as sepsis, hemorrhage, systemic inflammatory response syndrome, and are at high risk for the development of IAH. An incidence study done on MICU patients receiving large-volume resuscitation showed that 85% of patients enrolled developed IAH with IAP > 12 mmHg, 33% developed IAP > 20 mmHg and 25% met the criteria for ACS. These patients had median fluid balance of +6.9 L and Acute Physiology and Chronic Health Evaluation II (APACHE II) score of 23. Thus, data emphasized the high incidence of IAH in MICU patients receiving large-volume resuscitation [10]. In another prospective multi-institutional study done in 15 ICUs, of 491 patients enrolled, IAH occurred in almost half of all the patients and was twice as common in mechanically ventilated patients compared to those who were breathing spontaneously The study revealed that intra-abdominal hypertension proportionally increased the 28 and 90-day mortality [11]. Given the prevalence of IAH/ACS and associated mortality, it is important to be vigilant regarding the ACS development in MICU, especially in patients receiving the large-volume resuscitation.

4. Etiology

The abdomen is a closed cavity surrounded by rigid (pelvic bones, rib cage, spine) and flexible borders (Visceral organs, abdominal wall, diaphragm). There is an extent to which abdominal girth can increase and after an extent, the girth does not increase and results in intra-abdominal hypertension and thus, progressing to abdominal compartment syndrome.

Risk factors for IAH and ACS development can be divided as follows **Table 2**:

Risk factors for IAH and ACS
1. Decrease in abdominal wall compliance Burn Eschars Rectus sheath hematoma Obesity (BMI > 30 kg/m2) Ascites Abdominal surgery Mechanical ventilation with high PEEP Prone positioning
2. Increase in intra-abdominal volume *2.1 Increase in intra-luminal volume* Fecal matter/air/fluid within the organs Intestinal/Gastric distention such as colonic pseudo-obstruction, ileus, gastroparesis Damage control laparotomy *2.2 Increase in extra-luminal content* Retroperitoneal tumor or hemorrhage Pancreatitis Abdominal abscess Hemo/Pneumoperitoneum Liver transplantation Peritoneal dialysis Peritonitis
3. Secondary ACS Large volume resuscitation (> 5 L fluids in 24 hours) Hypothermia (core temperature less than 33 degree Celsius) Acidosis (pH < 7.2) Massive blood transfusion (>10 PRBC in 24 hrs) Coagulopathy (platelets <55,000 or prothrombin time > 15 secs or INR >1.5) Sepsis Major burns

Table 2.
Risk factors predisposing to IAH and ACS [12].

5. Pathophysiology

Like any other compartment syndrome, an increase in IAH, causes the decrease in perfusion of the contents within the abdominal cavity due to increased venous resistance, causing decreased capillary perfusion. However, IAH is an area of particular significance given the multi-systemic effect involving cardiac, pulmonary, and renal systems. Patients with underlying cardiomyopathy, renal insufficiency, pulmonary diseases are at high risk of decompensation [13].

5.1 Cardiovascular

Increase in IAP causes cephalad movement of the diaphragm leading to increased intrathoracic pressure. This phenomenon results in the following:

Decrease venous return: Increase in IAP, increases the pressure in the IVC and with the cephalad motion of the diaphragm, the thoracic inlet of the IVC constricts; thus, decreasing the venous return and the preload, thereby, affecting a component of cardiac output. Decreased venous return increases the hydrostatic pressure in lower extremities resulting in peripheral edema and increased risk for development of deep vein thrombosis [14].

Increase SVR: Increase in IAP causes increased pressure in systemic and aortic vasculature and also, increase pulmonary vascular resistance secondary to increased intrathoracic pressure. These factors thus increase SVR and thereby, decreasing the cardiac output [15].

Impaired cardiac function: Elevation of the diaphragm and increased intrathoracic pressure caused by IAH also causes cardiac compression, thus, decreasing ventricular compliance and contractility.

In conclusion, the MAP is affected by both SVR and Cardiac output. In absence of severe IAH, SVR increases, and cardiac output decreases (due to decreased preload). Thus, MAP remains stable despite a decrease in both preload and cardiac output. However, in patients with decreased intravascular volume or with poor cardiac function, even a mild to moderate increase in IAP can result in decreasing MAP. Therefore, preload augmentation with volume resuscitation appears to be beneficial to compensate for the increasing systemic vascular resistance. In ventilated patients, high PEEP or auto-PEEP can further decrease the venous return and thus, are also at risk of decompensation at the lower elevation of IAP.

5.2 Pulmonary

An increase in the IAP compresses the lung parenchyma by direct transmission of IAP and cephalad deviation of the diaphragm. Compression of lung parenchyma thus results in atelectasis, which results in increasing shunting of the blood and causes ventilation-perfusion mismatch. The atelectatic lung is also at higher risk for infection. In mechanically ventilated patients, increased IAP causes the peak inspiratory pressure and mean airway pressure to increase, thus causing the alveolar barotrauma. These patients also have decreased chest wall compliance and spontaneous tidal volume, causing hypoxemia and hypercarbia, which are the clinical features of ACS [16].

5.3 Renal

IAH significantly decreases the renal function and thus urine output by significantly affecting the renal blood flow. In comparison with superior mesenteric and celiac blood flow, studies have shown preferential decrease in renal blood flow with elevated IAP [17]. IAH results in renal arterial constriction and an increase in renal venous resistance, thus causing decrease in the venous drainage from the kidney. Secondarily, a decrease in cardiac output also results in activation of the renin-angiotensin-aldosterone system, thus causing renal arterial vasoconstriction. As mentioned above an increase in IAP affects the filtration gradient and thus, resulting in a net decrease in urine output. A study has shown development of oliguria at IAP of approximately 15 mmHg, whereas elevation of IAP to 30 mmHg results in anuria [18].

5.4 Gastrointestinal system

The gut is most sensitive to increased IAP. It affects the gut in the following ways:

Decreasing mesenteric blood flow: Mesenteric blood flow is decreased at IAP as low as 10 mmHg. A study showed 43% decrease in the celiac artery blood flow and 69% decrease in superior mesenteric artery blood flow when IAP is elevated to 40 mmHg. This is accentuated by shock and hypotension [17].

Compressing mesenteric veins: IAH compresses mesenteric veins in the intestinal wall causing impaired venous flow from the intestine and thus, causing intestinal edema. This edema in turn causes an elevation in the IAP, thus initiating a vicious cycle. This results in worsened hypoperfusion leading to elevation of lactic acid and intestinal ischemia.

Loss of intestinal mucosa: Gut hypoperfusion results in the loss of protective intestinal mucosal barrier, leading to gut bacterial translocation and results, in sepsis with multi-organ failure [19].

5.5 Hepatic

Elevation in IAP causes decreased hepatic arterial flow and increases the portal venous and hepatic venous resistance, thus, resulting in decreased microcirculatory blood flow in the liver. This results in decreased mitochondrial function and production of ATPs. Overall, the liver's capacity to clear lactic acid decreases. This has been seen at IAP elevation to as low as 10 mmHg in presence of normal cardiac output and MAP [20].

5.6 Central nervous system

Elevation in IAP causes increase in intracranial pressure (ICP) by decreasing the lumbar venous plexus blood flow and decreasing the cerebral venous outflow. Overall increase in partial pressure of carbon dioxide results in cerebral venous constriction resulting in increased ICP This, in turn, decreases the cerebral perfusion pressure and function [21].

5.7 Abdominal wall

Increased IAP can cause a decrease in blood flow to the abdominal wall, leading to wall ischemia and edema. Rectus sheath blood flow decreases in proportion to increase in the intra-abdominal pressure. It decreases by approximately 58% from baseline with IAP as low as 10 mmHg. This further reduces the abdominal wall compliance and exacerbates the IAH [22].

6. Clinical presentation

Early identification of IAH is imperative to prevent further progression to ACS. Most patients with ACS are critically ill and unable to express the symptoms, therefore, identifying the signs of IAH or developing ACS is very important.

Signs of ACS
• Abdominal distention and elevated IAP
• Oliguria refractory to volume resuscitation
• Hypoxia
• Hypercarbia
• Increased peak inspiratory pressure and PEEP
• Refractory metabolic acidosis
• Elevated ICP

Table 3.
Clinical signs of abdominal compartment syndrome [23].

6.1 Signs of abdominal compartment syndrome

Intraabdominal hypertension through its delirious effect on multi-organ system including kidney, lungs and cardiovascular system results in following clinical entities as mentioned in **Table 3** [23]. These clinical signs are seen commonly in critically ill patients having multiple comorbidities. Thus, it is very important to measure IAP at early stage and have high suspicion for ACS.

6.2 Imaging findings

These are not diagnostic for ACS, however, can be used as signs for early identification for developing abdominal compartment syndrome. Chest X-ray significant for elevated hemidiaphragm, pulmonary atelectasis and decreased lung volumes. CT scan findings are consistent with abdominal distention, tense infiltration of retroperitoneum out of proportion to the retroperitoneal disease, extrinsic compression of IVC or renal displacement, bowel wall thickening [24].

7. IAP measurement

In multiple prospective studies, the sensitivity of clinical examination in the diagnosis of IAH is only 40–60% [25, 26]. Abdomen being a hollow cavity filled with viscera, IAP can be measured by measuring the pressure within various viscera. However, IAP is typically measured via trans-bladder pressure measurement as recommended by the World Society of Abdominal Compartment Syndrome (WSACS) in 2006 due to ease of measurement [27]. Other ways to measure IAP include manometry from the abdominal drain, measuring pressure from central venous catheter inserted into inferior vena cava, measuring pressure via nasogastric tube, measuring rectal/uterine pressure [28]. Advanced modalities such as measuring abdominal wall thickness via ultrasound are also currently being investigated.

7.1 Intravesical pressure

Measurement of intravesical pressure has evolved over the years to decrease complications including the need for repeat measurements, urinary tract infection, and to decrease the incidence of needlestick injuries. The most common technique used is as follows:

- A three-way stopcock is used to decrease the number of times an aspiration port is accessed.

- A saline infusion set with 1000 ml normal saline bag is inserted in the first stopcock.
- A 50 ml syringe is attached to the 2nd stopcock.
- The third stopcock is attached to the pressure transducer and it is zeroed at a point where the mid-axillary line crosses the iliac crest.
- The urine drainage port of the foley is clamped.
- Instill 25 ml normal saline at room temperature into the bladder. Given that this normal saline can also result in detrusor muscle contraction and falsely increased the measured IAP, it is advisable to wait 30–60 seconds after saline administration to measure the pressure. Also, the patient should be in the complete supine position with a measurement done at end-expiration to ensure no abdominal muscle contraction is present. The measurement is done after the stopcocks to the pressure transducer is opened.

Although, intravesical pressure measurement is the gold standard to measure the intra-abdominal pressure, it has many technical difficulties. Though the evolution of technique has decreased the risk of needlestick injuries, this technique still is cumbersome, intermittent and carries potential risk of urinary tract infection. Most of the ventilated patients in MICU have head of bed elevated to prevent aspiration risk and studies have shown that the intravesical pressure increases significantly even with mild head of bed elevation [29].

7.2 Intra-gastric pressure

This method involves measurement of the pressure within the stomach using the nasogastric tube. It can be used when the patient does not have a foley catheter or intravesical pressure measurement is not possible due to bladder trauma, pelvic hematoma, peritoneal adhesions or neurogenic bladder. The use of tonometer to measure the intragastric pressure has been validated and showed good correlation with the IAP [30]. However, the IAP measured via nasogastric tube is affected by the migrating motor complex and the effects of enteral tube feeding on the IAP measurement are still unknown. The intra-gastric pressure measurement can also be used to monitor continuous intra-abdominal pressure. The most advanced method involves the air-pouch system where the tip of the nasogastric tube contains a pressure transducer which can automatically calibrate every hour and provides continuous intra-abdominal pressure measurement, however, this method is not validated in humans yet.

7.3 Inferior vena cava pressure

IVC catheter placed via femoral cannulation can be connected to the pressure transducer to provide IVC pressure measurement. A study validating the indirect methods of IAP measurement in rabbits showed good correlation of IVC and transvesical pressure with direct intraperitoneal pressure measurements. However, IVC catheter are associated with increased risk of infection and sepsis. A multicenter observational study showed that femoral vein pressure has good correlation with the IAP when intra-abdominal pressure is >20 mmHg and can be used as a surrogate to bladder pressure, thus, allowing continuous measurement of IAP [31].

7.4 Rectal and uterine pressure

Rectal and transvaginal pressure measurement is less practical given the pressure can be affected by the residual fecal mass or gynecological bleeding. Both these techniques have not been validated in the ICU setting [32].

8. Management

Management of ACS involves early recognition of IAH and/or end-organ failure and prompt interventions. It has been outlined by WSACS as shown in **Figures 1** and **2**. Management can be divided into medical and surgical interventions.

8.1 Non-surgical management

Non-surgical measures include decreasing the IAP by decreasing the content within the visceral organs that might be causing the IAH. Ileus is a common post-abdominal surgical complication and is also common amongst patients receiving large volume resuscitation, in patients with peritonitis, electrolyte imbalance and those receiving narcotic medications. These factors are independently associated to increase risk for IAH/ACS. Thus, treating ileus by nasogastric suction and rectal suction, use of prokinetic agents, colonoscopic decompression, and frequent enemas helps to decrease IAP by decreasing the volume of intra-luminal contents.

In patients where extra-luminal factors are leading to elevated IAH, alleviating the cause is most advisable to improve the abdominal wall compliance. If any space-occupying lesion is contributing to the IAH, thorough investigation including Ultrasound and CT scan should be done to identify the nature of space occupying lesion (SOL) and if indicated, either percutaneous drainage or surgical removal of the SOL can help with reducing the IAP. If ascites is contributing to the IAH, then

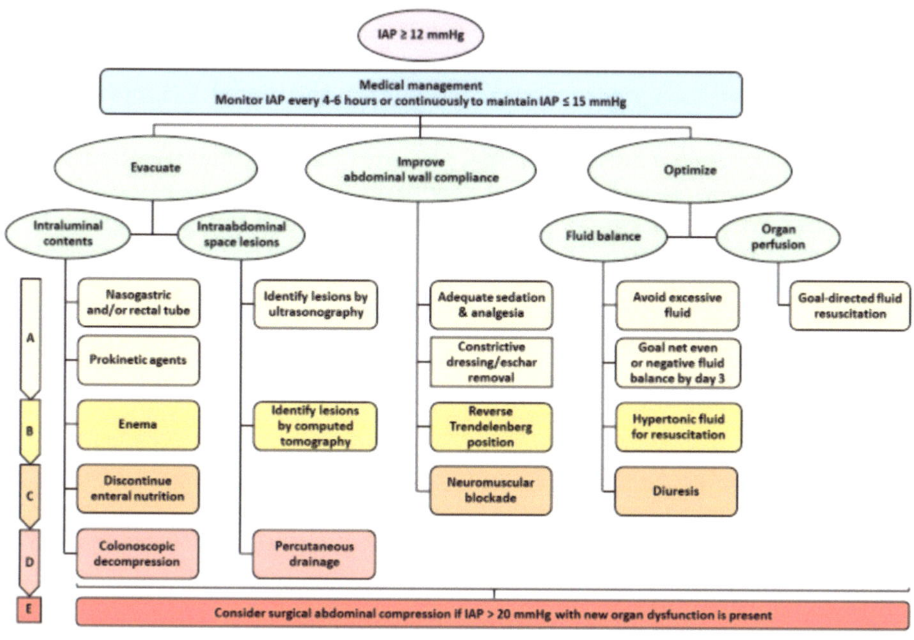

Figure 1.
Medical management for intra-abdominal hypertension [27].

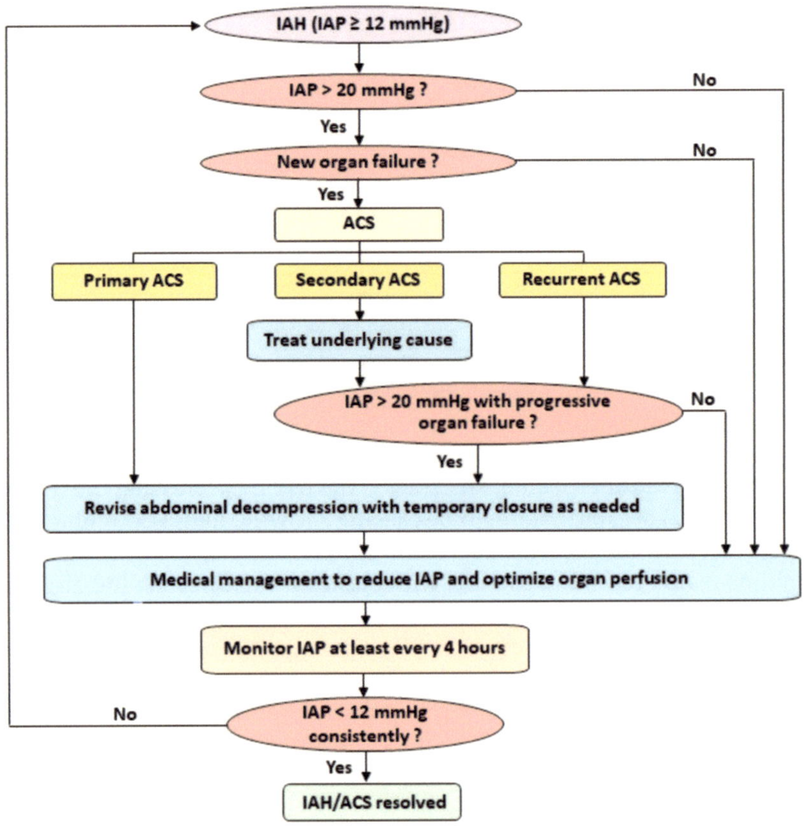

Figure 2.
Evaluation and management of abdominal compartment syndrome [4].

therapeutic paracentesis can help. However, in patients with progressive IAH or not responding to therapeutic paracentesis, continuous percutaneous drainage guided by Ultrasound or CT scan should be considered. Studies have shown that continuous percutaneous drainage decreases the rate of open abdominal decompression in 81% of the patients treated. However, if percutaneous drain fails to drain at least 1 L of fluid and decrease the intra-abdominal pressure by at least 9 mmHg in first four hours, the likelihood for requirement of surgical decompression increases [33].

Abdominal compliance can also be improved by adequate sedation and analgesia, removal of constrictive dressing, and eschars. Supine positioning or reverse Trendelenburg position also helps alleviate the abdominal muscle contracture. Low evidence is available but neuromuscular blockade should be considered per WSACS guidelines [27].

Managing the volume status of the patient is equally important, as hypovolemia can further exacerbate the effects of IAH and the large volume resuscitation can also similarly be shown as a predictive factor for progression to ACS. Thus, it's important to judge the volume status of the patient and maintain euvolemia. Hemodynamic monitoring is advisable for judicious administration of fluids. Recent study in burn patients receiving large volume resuscitation has shown that hypertonic saline or colloid solution effectively decreases the risk for developing IAH/ACS [34].

Despite adequate fluid resuscitation, some patients with IAH/ACS develop total body fluid overload secondary to capillary leakage and excessive third spacing with significant elevation in IAP [35]. Diuretics are generally contraindicated as these patients are intravascularly volume depleted. However, once these patients become hemodynamically stable with resolution of shock, diuretics along with colloid administration helps to the fluid from the third space. Continuous renal replacement therapy to remove excess fluid judiciously and increase abdominal wall compliance can also help decrease the IAP However, it's important to ensure that intra-vascular volume is adequately maintained for appropriate organ perfusion and avoidance of multi-organ failure development secondary to inadequate perfusion.

8.2 Surgical management

When the non-surgical methods fail to consistently decrease the IAP, surgical abdominal decompression via laparotomy is the treatment of choice. Decompressive laparotomy results in a decrease in intra-abdominal volume and thus decreases the IAP. Delay in surgical depression in surgical and non-surgical patients is associated with increased mortality [36]. There is also an increased risk of ischemia–reperfusion syndrome especially in patients with significantly high IAP for a prolonged period. Abdominal laparotomy with negative peritoneal pressure therapy is preferred given that it improves visceral perfusion and also decreases bacterial translocation. In multiple studies, surgical decompression has been shown to decrease IAP and improve respiratory, cardiac, and renal function [37]. However, studies on the mortality related to ACS requiring decompressive laparotomy are inconclusive as there is a significant difference in when the decision to do decompression is made by the intensivist based on their specialty. Studies have shown that medical intensivists prefer diuresis and dialysis more and take double the time than surgical intensivists to decide on decompressive laparotomy. Surgical decompression, though a life-saving procedure, has significant morbidity and mortality associated with it. In a study, three out of four patients of severe acute pancreatitis who underwent surgical decompression died and two of them from uncontrollable retroperitoneal hemorrhage [38].

Decompressive laparotomy can result in excess loss of fluids from the exposed tissue resulting in exsanguination or can result in a large ventral hernia or fistula [39]. The open abdomen also increases risk for bacterial translocation and sepsis. Thus, steps should be taken to close the abdomen as soon as possible with most surgeons planning staged closure every 48 hours. Continued manometric measurement of IAP even after abdominal closure is necessary.

9. Prognosis

ACS is associated with high mortality and hence, it's imperative to identify the early signs of intra-abdominal hypertension. Presence of IAH on day 1 of ICU is not an independent risk factor for mortality, however, occurrence and persistence of IAH during the ICU stay has significant associated with mortality [40]. Studies have shown that mortality increases proportionally with abdominal hypertension. A study showed 45.1% mortality in ACS patients compared to 21% mortality in patients with increased IAP [41]. Most common cause leading to death includes sepsis and multi-organ failure.

10. Conclusion

Intra-abdominal hypertension and abdominal compartment syndrome are prevalent amongst critically ill medical patients and associated with high mortality.

Thus, medical staff should have a high suspicion of ACS in critically ill patients. Large volume resuscitation should be rationalized, and early surgical decompression must be considered if indicated.

Conflict of interest

The authors declare no conflict of interest.

Author details

Kejal Gandhi[1], Pahnwat Taweesedt[2], Munish Sharma[2], Dweep Barbhaya[1] and Salim Surani[3*]

1 Georgetown University/Medstar Washington Hospital Center, Washington, DC, USA

2 Corpus Christi Medical Center, Texas, USA

3 Christus Spohn Hospital Corpus Christi – Memorial, Corpus Christi, Texas, USA

*Address all correspondence to: srsurani@hotmail.com

References

[1] Bailey J, Shapiro MJ. Abdominal compartment syndrome. Crit Care [Internet]. 2000;4(1):23. Available from: https://doi.org/10.1186/cc646

[2] De Keulenaer BL, De Waele JJ, Powell B, Malbrain M. What is normal intra-abdominal pressure and how is it affected by positioning, body mass and positive end-expiratory pressure? Intensive Care Med. 2009;35(6):969-976.

[3] Cheatham ML, White MW, Sagraves SG, Johnson JL, Block EFJ. Abdominal Perfusion Pressure: A Superior Parameter in the Assessment of Intra-abdominal Hypertension. J Trauma Acute Care Surg [Internet]. 2000;49(4). Available from: https://journals.lww.com/jtrauma/Fulltext/2000/10000/Abdominal_Perfusion_Pressure__A_Superior_Parameter.8.aspx

[4] Cheatham ML, Malbrain MLNG, Kirkpatrick A, Sugrue M, Parr M, De Waele J, et al. Results from the International Conference of Experts on Intra-abdominal Hypertension and Abdominal Compartment Syndrome. II. Recommendations. Intensive Care Med [Internet]. 2007;33(6):951-62. Available from: https://doi.org/10.1007/s00134-007-0592-4

[5] Malbrain MLNG, De laet IE, De Waele JJ, Kirkpatrick AW. Intra-abdominal hypertension: Definitions, monitoring, interpretation and management. Best Pract Res Clin Anaesthesiol [Internet]. 2013;27(2):249-270. Available from: http://www.sciencedirect.com/science/article/pii/S152168961300044X

[6] Malbrain MLNG, De Keulenaer BL, Oda J, De Waele J, Roberts DJ, Kirkpatrick AW, et al. Intra-abdominal hypertension and abdominal compartment syndrome in burns, obesity, pregnancy, and general medicine. Anaesthesiol Intensive Ther. 2015;47(3):228-240.

[7] Dalfino L, Tullo L, Donadio I, Malcangi V, Brienza N. Intra-abdominal hypertensionand acute renal failurein critically ill patients. Intensive Care Med [Internet]. 2008;34(4):707-13. Available from: https://doi.org/10.1007/s00134-007-0969-4

[8] Tons C, Schachtrupp A, Rau M, Mumme T, Schumpelick V. Abdominal compartment syndrome: avoidance and treatment. Der Chir. 2000;71(8):918-926.

[9] Rajasurya V, Surani S. Abdominal compartment syndrome: Often overlooked conditions in medical intensive care units. World J Gastroenterol. 2020;26(3):266.

[10] Daugherty EL, Liang H, Taichman D, Hansen-Flaschen J, Fuchs BD. Abdominal Compartment Syndrome Is Common in Medical Intensive Care Unit Patients Receiving Large-Volume Resuscitation. J Intensive Care Med [Internet]. 2007 Sep 1;22(5):294-9. Available from: https://doi.org/10.1177/0885066607305247

[11] Reintam Blaser A, Regli A, De Keulenaer B, Kimball EJ, Starkopf L, Davis WA, et al. Incidence, Risk Factors, and Outcomes of Intra-Abdominal Hypertension in Critically Ill Patients-A Prospective Multicenter Study (IROI Study). Crit Care Med. 2019 Apr;47(4):535-542.

[12] Malbrain MLNG, De laet IE. Intra-Abdominal Hypertension: Evolving Concepts. Clin Chest Med [Internet]. 2009;30(1):45-70. Available from: http://www.sciencedirect.com/science/article/pii/S0272523108000919

[13] Papavramidis TS, Marinis AD, Pliakos I, Kesisoglou I, Papavramidou N.

Abdominal compartment syndrome–Intra-abdominal hypertension: Defining, diagnosing, and managing. J Emergencies, Trauma Shock. 2011;4(2):279.

[14] Kashtan J, Green JF, Parsons EQ, Holcroft JW. Hemodynamic effects of increased abdominal pressure. J Surg Res [Internet]. 1981;30(3):249-255. Available from: http://www.sciencedirect.com/science/article/pii/0022480481901566

[15] Luca A, Cirera I, García-Pagán JC, Feu F, Pizcueta P, Bosch J, et al. Hemodynamic effects of acute changes in intra-abdominal pressure in patients with cirrhosis. Gastroenterology. 1993 Jan;104(1):222-227.

[16] Pelosi P, Quintel M, Malbrain MLNG. Effect of intra-abdominal pressure on respiratory mechanics. Acta Clin Belg. 2007;62 Suppl 1:78-88.

[17] Barnes GE, Laine GA, Giam PY, Smith EE, Granger HJ. Cardiovascular responses to elevation of intra-abdominal hydrostatic pressure. Am J Physiol Integr Comp Physiol [Internet]. 1985 Feb 1;248(2):R208-13. Available from: https://doi.org/10.1152/ajpregu.1985.248.2.R208

[18] Richards WO, Scovill W, Shin B, Reed W. Acute renal failure associated with increased intra-abdominal pressure. Ann Surg. 1983 Feb;197(2):183-187.

[19] De Laet IE, Malbrain M. Current insights in intra-abdominal hypertension and abdominal compartment syndrome. Med intensiva. 2007;31(2):88-99.

[20] Diebel LN, Wilson RF, Dulchavsky SA, Saxe J. Effect of increased intra-abdominal pressure on hepatic arterial, portal venous, and hepatic microcirculatory blood flow. J Trauma [Internet]. 1992 Aug;33(2):279—82; discussion 282—3. Available from: https://doi.org/10.1097/00005373-199208000-00019

[21] Bloomfield GL, Ridings PC, Blocher CR, Marmarou A, Sugerman HJ. Effects of Increased Intra-abdominal Pressure upon Intracranial and Cerebral Perfusion Pressure before and after Volume Expansion. J Trauma Acute Care Surg [Internet]. 1996;40(6). Available from: https://journals.lww.com/jtrauma/Fulltext/1996/06000/Effects_of_Increased_Intra_abdominal_Pressure_upon.12.aspx

[22] Diebel, L., Saxe, J. M., & Dulchavsky S. Effects of Intra-Abdominal Pressure on Abdominal Wall Blood Flow. Am Surg [Internet]. 1992;58(9):573-576. Available from: https://corescholar.libraries.wright.edu/surg/134

[23] Ivatury RR, Diebel L, Porter JM, Simon RJ. INTRA-ABDOMINAL HYPERTENSION AND THE ABDOMINAL COMPARTMENT SYNDROME. Surg Clin North Am [Internet]. 1997;77(4):783-800. Available from: http://www.sciencedirect.com/science/article/pii/S0039610905705843

[24] Pickhardt PJ, Shimony JS, Heiken JP, Buchman TG, Fisher AJ. The abdominal compartment syndrome: CT findings. AJR Am J Roentgenol. 1999 Sep;173(3):575-579.

[25] Kirkpatrick AW, Brenneman FD, McLean RF, Rapanos T, Boulanger BR. Is clinical examination an accurate indicator of raised intra-abdominal pressure in critically injured patients? Can J Surg [Internet]. 2000 Jun;43(3):207-211. Available from: https://pubmed.ncbi.nlm.nih.gov/10851415

[26] Blaser AR, Sarapuu S, Tamme K, Starkopf J. Expanded Measurements of Intra-Abdominal Pressure Do Not Increase the Detection Rate of Intra-Abdominal Hypertension: A Single-Center Observational Study*. Crit Care Med [Internet]. 2014;42(2). Available from: https://journals.lww.com/ccmjournal/Fulltext/2014/02000/Expanded_Measurements_of_Intra_Abdominal_Pressure.18.aspx

[27] Kirkpatrick AW, Roberts DJ, De Waele J, Jaeschke R, Malbrain MLNG, De Keulenaer B, et al. Intra-abdominal hypertension and the abdominal compartment syndrome: updated consensus definitions and clinical practice guidelines from the World Society of the Abdominal Compartment Syndrome. Intensive Care Med [Internet]. 2013;39(7):1190-206. Available from: https://doi.org/10.1007/s00134-013-2906-z

[28] Malbrain MLNG. Different techniques to measure intra-abdominal pressure (IAP): time for a critical re-appraisal. Appl Physiol intensive care Med. 2006;105-119.

[29] Cheatham ML, De Waele JJ, De Laet I, De Keulenaer B, Widder S, Kirkpatrick AW, et al. The impact of body position on intra-abdominal pressure measurement: A multicenter analysis*. Crit Care Med [Internet]. 2009;37(7). Available from: https://journals.lww.com/ccmjournal/Fulltext/2009/07000/The_impact_of_body_position_on_intra_abdominal.8.aspx

[30] Sugrue M, Buist MD, Lee A, Sanchez DJ, Hillman KM. Intra-abdominal pressure measurement using a modified nasogastric tube: description and validation of a new technique. Intensive Care Med [Internet]. 1994;20(8):588-590. Available from: http://europepmc.org/abstract/MED/7706574

[31] Howard AE, Regli A, Litton E, Malbrain MM, Palermo A-M, De Keulenaer BL. Can Femoral Venous Pressure be Used as an Estimate for Standard Vesical Intra-Abdominal Pressure Measurement? Anaesth Intensive Care [Internet]. 2016 Nov 1;44(6):704-11. Available from: https://doi.org/10.1177/0310057X1604400604

[32] Sugrue M, De Waele J, De Keulenaer BL, Roberts DJ, Malbrain MLNG. A user's guide to intra-abdominal pressure measurement. Anaesthesiol Intensive Ther. 2015;47(3):241-251.

[33] Cheatham ML, Safcsak K. Percutaneous catheter decompression in the treatment of elevated intraabdominal pressure. Chest. 2011 Dec;140(6):1428-1435.

[34] O'Mara MS, Slater H, Goldfarb IW, Caushaj PF. A prospective, randomized evaluation of intra-abdominal pressures with crystalloid and colloid resuscitation in burn patients. J Trauma. 2005 May;58(5):1011-1018.

[35] Cordemans C, De laet I, Van Regenmortel N, Schoonheydt K, Dits H, Huber W, et al. Fluid management in critically ill patients: the role of extravascular lung water, abdominal hypertension, capillary leak, and fluid balance. Ann Intensive Care [Internet]. 2012;2(1):S1. Available from: https://doi.org/10.1186/2110-5820-2-S1-S1

[36] Mentula P, Hienonen P, Kemppainen E, Puolakkainen P, Leppäniemi A. Surgical Decompression for Abdominal Compartment Syndrome in Severe Acute Pancreatitis. Arch Surg [Internet]. 2010 Aug 1;145(8):764-9. Available from: https://doi.org/10.1001/archsurg.2010.132

[37] Rogers WK, Garcia L. Intraabdominal Hypertension, Abdominal Compartment Syndrome,

and the Open Abdomen. Chest [Internet]. 2018;153(1):238-250. Available from: http://www.sciencedirect.com/science/article/pii/S0012369217313193

[38] De Waele JJ, Hoste E, Blot SI, Decruyenaere J, Colardyn F. Intra-abdominal hypertension in patients with severe acute pancreatitis. Crit Care [Internet]. 2005;9(4):R452. Available from: https://doi.org/10.1186/cc3754

[39] De Waele JJ, Kimball E, Malbrain M, Nesbitt I, Cohen J, Kaloiani V, et al. Decompressive laparotomy for abdominal compartment syndrome. Br J Surg. 2016;103(6):709.

[40] Malbrain MLNG, Chiumello D, Pelosi P, Bihari D, Innes R, Ranieri VM, et al. Incidence and prognosis of intraabdominal hypertension in a mixed population of critically ill patients: a multiple-center epidemiological study. Crit Care Med. 2005;33(2):315-322.

[41] Parsak CK, Seydaoglu G, Sakman G, Acarturk TO, Karakoc E, Hanta I, et al. Abdominal Compartment Syndrome: Current Problems and New Strategies. World J Surg [Internet]. 2008;32(1):13-9. Available from: https://doi.org/10.1007/s00268-007-9286-x

Chapter 7

Compartment Syndrome Related to Patient Positioning in the Surgical Treatment of Urolithiasis

Inés Laso-García, Fernando Arias-Fúnez, Gemma Duque-Ruiz, David Díaz-Pérez, Alberto Artiles-Medina and Javier Burgos-Revilla

Abstract

The incidence of urolithiasis is progressively increasing worldwide, as is the surgical treatment of urinary stones. The most frequent surgery for urolithiasis is ureterorenoscopy, which is performed in the lithotomy position. This position is also used in the endoscopic approach to bladder stones. Lateral decubitus is rarely used in the treatment of urinary stones. In the case of complex kidney stones, the gold standard treatment is percutaneous nephrolithotomy. This surgery has traditionally been performed in the prone position. However, the use of the supine (Valdivia) position is increasing in recent times. Furthermore, the Galdakao-modified supine Valdivia position has been widely used for percutaneous nephrolithotomy since it was described by Ibarluzea et al. in 2007. Treatment of kidney and ureteral stones simultaneously is allowed in both supine positions. In addition, they allow the removal of encrusted stents and the easy placement of double J stents and, in the case of the Galdakao-modified supine Valdivia position, percutaneous nephrostomies. Compartment syndrome is a rare complication in the lithotomy position, but scarcely described in the supine position. This especially applies to the Galdakao-modified supine Valdivia position, in which the lower limbs are in moderate flexion, with the ipsilateral lower limb in a slightly lower position relative to the other. This complication can lead to skin necrosis, myoglobinuric renal failure, amputation, permanent neuromuscular dysfunction, and even death. Risk factors include Body Mass Index, male gender, obesity, increased muscle mass, peripheral vascular disease (advanced age, hypertension, hyperlipidemia and diabetes mellitus), height, lack of operative experience, significant bleeding during surgery, hypothermia, acidemia, combination general-spinal anesthesia, prolonged surgical time, systemic hypotension, ASA (American Society of Anesthesiologists) class or vasoconstrictor drugs. Therefore, compartment syndrome of the leg is a potentially devastating complication that must be suspected and treated through early decompression of the compartment by four compartment fasciotomy. Preventive measures reduce the incidence of this condition.

Keywords: lithiasis, percutaneous nephrolithotomy, Galdakao-modified supine valdivia position, complications, compartment syndrome

1. Introduction

1.1 Urolithiasis

Urinary lithiasis is a disease known since ancient times, characterized by the formation of urinary stones (**Figure 1**). The prevalence of lithiasis in the population in 1913 has been estimated to be 1–2%, and a progressive increase has been found to 2.7% in 1985. [1] An article studying the evolution of the prevalence in a 25-year-period, showed an annual increase in stone formation. The prevalence of lithiasis in population has grown even more in recent years. [2] The incidence of lithiasis in the United States doubled in a 4 year-period. [3]

Furthermore, Scales et al. described a prevalence of almost 9% of the population. [4] Nevertheless, it has been observed a variation according to the country studied: 1–5% in Asia, 5–9% in Europe, 13% in North America and 20% in Saudi Arabia. [5]

In recent years, in the United Kingdom, a 63% increase in hospitalization episodes associated with urolithiasis has been observed. [6] The number of extracorporeal shock wave lithotripsy has increased from 14,491 in 2000 to 822,402 in 2010. There has been an increase of 127% in the number of ureteroscopies. The acts aimed at treating urinary lithiasis have increased compared to other urological activities. In 2010, shock wave lithotripsy was performed with the same frequency as transurethral resection of the prostate or transurethral resection of the bladder. More ureteroscopies were performed than nephrectomies, prostatectomies, and cystectomies combined; and more percutaneous nephrolithectomies than cystectomies. [7] Therefore, the surgical treatment of urolithiasis is of great clinical relevance.

1.2 Surgical positions in urological surgery and urolithiasis

The most frequent surgery for urolithiasis is ureterorenoscopy, which is performed in the lithotomy (Lloyd-Davies) position. This position is also used in the endoscopic approach to bladder stones.

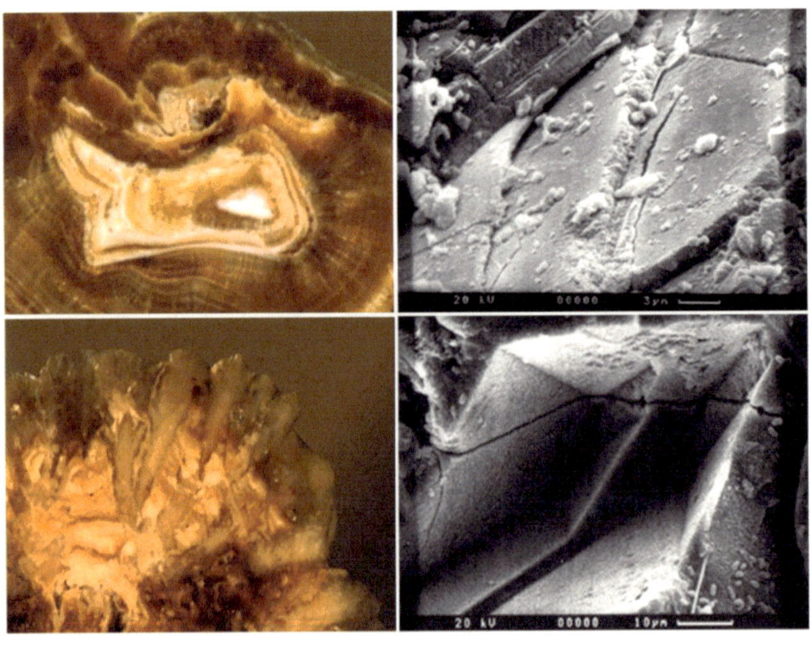

Figure 1.
Calcium oxalate lithiasis: conventional microscope and scanning electron microscope.

Percutaneous nephrolithectomy is currently the treatment of choice for complex renal and renoureteral stones (for example, staghorn lithiasis, **Figure 2**). This surgery has traditionally been performed in the prone position, but in recent years the number of urologists who perform it in the supine position (Valdivia Position) has increased. [8–11]

Ibarluzea et al. described the Galdakao-modified supine Valdivia position in 2007, and it has been widely used for percutaneous nephrolithotomy since then. [11] Treatment of kidney and ureteral stones simultaneously is allowed in both supine positions. In addition, they allow the removal of encrusted stents and the easy placement of double J stents and, in the case of the Galdakao-modified supine Valdivia position, percutaneous nephrostomies. Unlike the prone position, the patient does not need to be relocated during surgery, shortening the operating time. In addition, it allows two surgeons to operate simultaneously.

1.3 The Galdakao-modified supine valdivia position for percutaneous nephrolithotomy

Occasionally, lower extremities are bandaged to prevent venous thrombosis. Once the patient is placed, retrograde pyelography is performed. The upper urinary tract is accessed through an X-ray and ultrasound guided puncture of the lower calyx. After Alken telescopic dilatation, an Amplatz sheath is placed to allow the passage of a nephroscope, reaching the upper urinary tract lumen.

Using the nephroscope and a retrograde flexible ureteroscope, the whole upper urinary tract can be managed, as decribed by Ibarluzea and Scoffone. [10, 11] This procedure is called Endoscope Combined IntraRenal Surgery (ECIRS).

Sources of lithiasis fragmentation, such as Holmium laser, as well as nitinol baskets, are used to remove the lithiasis. If the stone is too complex, this process can be lengthy, or even ineffective, in treating the entire stone.

1.4 Compartment syndrome related to patient positioning

The position in which a patient is placed, and the duration for which it is maintained, are key factors in the development of well-leg compartment syndrome.

Acute compartment syndrome of the extremities rarely develops in the supine position, commonly used in urologic open surgeries, such as cystolithotomy. Lateral decubitus position is rarely used in the treatment of urolithiasis. Laparoscopic

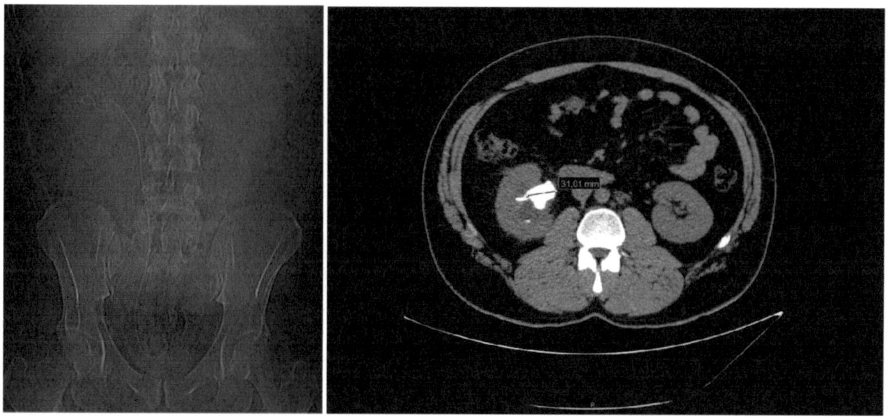

Figure 2.
Right kidney staghorn lithiasis.

pyelolithectomy would be one of the examples. General complications of lateral decubitus positioning are similar to those found with the supine position.

It has been described that lithotomy position, in general surgical, urological and orthopedic patients, is associated with changes in intracompartmental pressure that may eventually develop a compartment syndrome, especially in prolonged surgeries. [12–15]

Well-leg compartment syndrome has also been described in patients placed in the hemilithotomy position. The majority of cases described in the literature have been lengthy procedures with surgical time greater than 5 h. [13]

Prolonged positioning in a steep Trendelenburg position during, for example, a laparoscopic prostatectomy, may cause hypoperfusion of the lower extremities, pressure marks, tissue injury, and even rhabdomyolysis. After long surgical procedures involving extreme positions, rhabdomyolysis from muscle ischemia has been observed. [16]

Acute compartment syndrome of the leg occurs following a rise in the pressure inside the muscle compartment. [16] A significant decrease in deep muscle mixed tissue oxygen saturation of calf muscles is observed, due to the combined effect of perfusion related factors, such as hydrostatic forces, blood and intra-abdominal pressure, which lead to tissue underperfusion. [17, 18]

A delay in the diagnosis and treatment of a compartment syndrome may lead to devastating outcomes for the patient. [19] It may lead to admission to an Intensive Care Unit and necessity of renal replacement therapy, multiple organ dysfunction syndrome, and even death.

Therefore, the suspicion of this syndrome in a patient who presents symptoms compatible with this adverse outcome, is essential to avoid further complications.

2. Epidemiology

Prolonged urological surgeries performed in the lithotomy or extreme Trendelemburg positions for the treatment of urolithiasis may rarely lead to well-leg compartment syndrome. [20] It is thought to be underreported in the literature, especially those with less severe clinical features. Moreover, it is generally misdiagnosed as other possible surgical complications, such as deep vein thrombosis or neuropraxia. [21, 22] In the lithotomy position, the estimated total rate is approximately 1: 3500. [17]

However, studies reporting on the compartment syndrome associated with the lithotomy position in the fields of general and gynecological surgeries are somewhat frequent [23] This complication has also been described in the literature regarding urological surgeries. [21] In some cases, the complication occurs in both extremities simultaneously. [24–26] This circumstance is often described in relation to the performance of a radical prostatectomy, either laparoscopic or robotic, in the extreme Trendelenburg position. [19, 27]

Nonetheless, the appearance of this complication is not frequent during a percutaneous nephrolithotomy. It has hardly been reported in both supine positions, in which the lower limbs present a more moderate flexion than in other endourological procedures. In the Galdakao-Modified Supine Valdivia Position, the patient is placed in a slightly different position from the classic lithotomy, with the lower limbs in moderate flexion, and with the ipsilateral lower limb in a slightly inferior position with respect to the other (**Figure 3**). [28] On the other hand, the appearance of acute abdominal compartment syndrome has already been described during the performance of a percutaneous nephrolithotomy. [29]

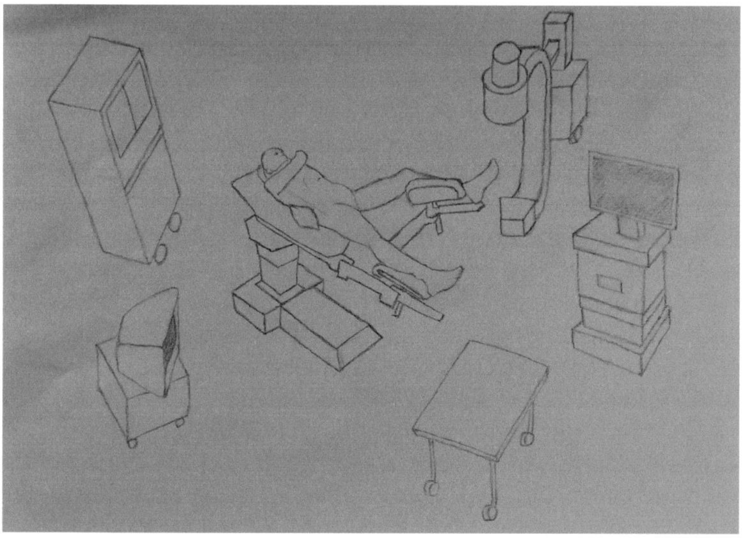

Figure 3.
The Galdakao-modified supine Valdivia position.

3. Etiology

Risk factors (**Table 1**) associated with the development of compartment syndrome reported include Body Mass Index (BMI), male gender, obesity, height, peripheral vascular disease (advanced age, hypertension, hyperlipidemia and

Related to the patient	Obesity
	Advanced age
	Hypertension
	Hyperlipidemia
	Diabetes Mellitus
	Height
	BMI
	Male sex
	ASA (American Society of Anesthesiologists) class
	Increased muscle bulk
Related to the surgery	Prolonged surgery time
	Systemic hypotension
	Acidemia
	Lack of operative experience
	Combined general-spinal anesthesia
	Hypothermia
	The use of vasoconstricting drugs
	Important bleeding during the surgery
	Wrapping elevated legs

Table 1.
Risk factors associated to the development of compartment syndrome.

diabetes mellitus), lack of operative experience, significant bleeding during surgery, hypothermia, acidemia, combination general-spinal anesthesia, prolonged surgical time, systemic hypotension, ASA (American Society of Anesthesiologists) class or vasoconstrictor drugs. Increased muscle bulk is associated with a tighter and less compliant compartment, and also with greater accumulation of toxic metabolites and free radicals. [17, 18, 21–23, 29–31]

The use of compressive leg wraps has been associated with well-leg compartment syndrome in some studies, [12] while in others a reduction in intracompartment pressure of the lower leg was observed with the use of external intermittent compression. [14]

4. Pathophysiology

Compartment syndromes can arise in any area of the body that has little or no capacity for tissue expansion, such as the abdomen, buttocks and hands.

The lower extremity has four main compartments, which are superficial posterior, deep posterior, anterior and lateral. Bone and inelastic fascial layers border the muscles and neurovascular structures. The following nerves traverse these compartments: the tibial and sural nerves, and the superficial and deep branches of the peroneal nerve. The compartment can be accommodated to a limited extent by the sheath. [16] Most commonly involved compartment is the anterior one. [21] As soon as legs are placed in the lithotomy position, the compartmental pressures begin to increase. [17] The height above the level of the heart at which the legs rise is crucial. [17, 18]

An increase in intracompartment pressure in the lithotomy position, with the use of support behind the calf or knee, has been described from 10.7 (SD 5.8) mmHg to 16.5 (SD 3.4) mmHg. [14] Circulation compromise occurs with increased tissue pressure within a closed osteofascial compartment. Compression of the calf produces local ischaemia through two mechanisms: by direct occlusion of the arterial blood flow and by indirect obstruction of the venous drainage. The weight of the limb itself, as well as the use of devices such as braces and cushions, produces greater compression. It should also be noted that operating personnel can cause more compression. [17]

The difference between capillary perfusion pressure and the interstitial fluid pressure determines tissue perfusion. When interstitial fluid pressure exceeds capillary perfusion pressure, capillary collapse and consequent ischemia of the muscles and nerves occurs. [32] It has two main implications: a decrease in the rates of both delivery of oxygenated arterial blood and drainage of deoxygenated venous blood. [17]

The integrity of the vascular endothelium is impaired by initial ischemia. Its capacity as a barrier to the movement of solute and serum disappears. Thus, a self-perpetuating cycle of ischaemia and tissue oedema begins. When the patient returns to the initial position, the compartment pressure may increase even further, producing a reperfusion injury. [16, 17] After 1 h of ischaemia, on restoring blood flow, through the release of prostaglandins and thromboxane, platelets are activated. This may predispose to deep vein thrombosis, which may increase venous pressure and therefore, compromise local blood flow. [18]

In addition, once reperfusion occurs, large amounts of toxic intracellular content are released into the bloodstream. They are the markers of rhabdomyolysis. [18] After surgery, serum creatine phosphokinase increases significantly, peaking at 18 hours. [19] The main pathophysiologic mechanisms involved in renal insufficiency from rhabdomyolysis are renal vasoconstriction, intraluminal cast formation, and direct myoglobin toxicity. [16]

5. Clinical features

5.1 Clinical findings

Once the patient is in the recovery room, in the immediate postoperative period, despite analgesic infusion, significant pain is reported in the lower extremity (a pain out of proportion). The limb appears oedematous and cyanotic, although the pedis pulses may be preserved. General inflammation of the leg and dorsal ankle flexion and toe mobility deficit is observed. In a more advanced stage, we may observe the absence of peripheral pulses. [24]

5.2 Intraoperative findings

Once the compartment fasciotomy has been performed, we can observe that only the deep compartments may be affected by ischemia. In this case, the muscle mass of the anterolateral compartment and the deep posteromedial compartment shows evidence of necrosis. Muscles show pale pink edema. Stimulation with an electric scapel shows absence of contractility. Correct tonality and contractility can be seen in the muscle mass of both superficial compartments if this occurs. When diagnosis and treatment are delayed, both deep and superficial masses are affected by ischemia.

6. Diagnosis

After lengthy surgeries, we must be aware of the possibility of the development of a compartment syndrome. Prompt diagnosis and treatment should be performed using a four-compartment fasciotomy to avoid serious and irreversible complications. [23]

The appearance of the following signs and symptoms must warn us: pink skin, presence of pulse, paresis of muscles, paraesthesia and a disproportionate pain, generally described by the patient as burning and deep. It is reproduced by passive stretching of the muscles of the compartment. The diagnosis is more difficult in unconscious and sedated patients.

On analysis, serum creatinine kinase activity is increased. We must bear in mind that the first signs are subtle and more often neurological. This is due to the fact that nonmyelinated type C sensory fibers are the tissues most sensitive to hypoxia. [21, 32] Therefore, a delay in the diagnosis should be considered with the use of epidural anesthesia, due to a masking effect. [21]

However, the definitive diagnosis is made by direct measurement of the compartmental pressure. Compartment pressure can be measured with different pressure catheters. These catheters have fine bore and their use is associated with minimal morbidity. [24] It can be measured by using a simple needle manometer, continuous infusion, wick catheter, slit catheter, or solid-state transducer method. [30] The indication for a fasciotomy is a value greater than 20–30 mmHg, although it may vary depending on the perfusion pressure and the clinical setting. [32]

We can use various non-invasive imaging techniques to determine intracompartment pressure, including laser Doppler flowmetry, ultrasonic devices, or near infrared spectroscopy. [16] These techniques might be particularly useful in pediatric patients, in whom invasive monitoring is not ideal. Near-infrared spectroscopy has proven useful in one-month-old infants. Nevertheless, both laser Doppler flowmetry and near-infrared spectroscopy may be more useful in chronic compartment syndrome, as they measure variations in muscle oxygenation. In acute compartment syndrome, changes may have already occurred at the time of measurement. Magnetic resonance imaging has limited utility in the diagnosis of acute compartment syndrome, as it can detect oedema and swelling, but only when the syndrome is well established, delaying the diagnosis.

In rhabdomyolysis, we can observe the presence of myoglobinuria in the absence of urinary erythrocytes. An increase in serum creatine phosphokinase activity is observed. Increased levels of other markers, such as phosphate, potassium, lactate dehydrogenase, aspartate, and alanine aminotransferase, may be seen in rhabdomyolysis. [17]

Venous thrombosis should be ruled out through Doppler ultrasound. Differential diagnoses include venous thrombosis and peripheral nerve or arterial injury.

It has to be taken into account that the limb may be capable of being saved up to 10–12 hours after the complication sets in.

7. Treatment

7.1 Surgical treatment

Regarding treatment (**Table 2**), early decompression of the compartment must be performed by an orthopedic surgeon, to avoid the self-perpetuating cycle of ischaemia and oedema.

Long incisions (20–25 cm) are made along the length of the leg. After that adequate and extensile incision, complete released of all involved compartment and preservation of vital structures is performed. All necrotic tissue is removed. Care should be taken to avoid the superficial peroneal nerve damage. The relief of pressure minimizes functional impairment, structural damage, and breaks the cycle of ischemia and edema, preventing additional devitalization of tissue and infection risk. [12]

If necessary, the four compartments are open, and if the muscles are under tension, the skin is left open, and approximated with vessel-loop temporarily. Only around 15% can be primarily closed without high compartment pressure.

Surgical treatment	If necessary, four compartments opening Long incisions (20–25 cm) along the length of the leg Complete release of all involved compartments Preservation of vital structures Necrotic tissue removal Avoidance of superficial peroneal nerve damage In muscles under tension: skin left open Use of moist dressings Skin incisions closing after a few days (for repeat irrigation and debridement)
Medical treatment	Adequate analgesia Early and aggressive fluid replacement Central venous monitoring Transferring to high dependency unit/intensive care therapy unit Adequately hydration (target urinary output of at least 0.5 ml/kg.) Use of mannitol (renal vasodilator effect, expands intravascular volume and decreases oxygen radicals) Urinary pH maintained as neutral as possible (avoidance urate and myoglobin precipitation): sodium bicarbonate or acetazolamide

Table 2.
Surgical and medical treatment of well-leg compartment syndrome.

Moist dressings are used the following days, and the skin incisions are usually closed after a few days or weeks with a non-absorbable (polypropylene) suture. There may be need for repeat irrigation and debridement before final wound closure. [17, 32]

Other options for the closure of fasciotomy wounds include split-thickness skin graft. It has been recommended the use of meshed split-thickness skin graft secured with foam vacuum suction dressing after excising all devitalized tissues. [24]

Pain is a major feature of compartment syndrome and adequate analgesia should be prescribed. [16]

7.2 Medical treatment

Creatine phosphokinase may reach values over 80,000 IU / L. In rhabdomyolysis, myoglobinuric renal failure develops, followed by multisystemic organ failure and possible death. Renal failure should be treated with early and aggressive fluid replacement, central venous monitoring and transfer to high dependency unit/ intensive care therapy unit.

Mean Arterial Pressure should be maintained over 65 mmHg. Patients should be adequately hydrated to achieve a target urinary output of at least 0.5 mL/Kg. [16] Mannitol may be used as it has a renal vasodilator effect. It also expands intravascular volume and decreases oxygen radicals. Urinary pH should be maintained as neutral as possible to avoid urate and myoglobin precipitation by alkalizing urine with sodium bicarbonate or acetazolamide. [21]

Wound infection is a potential complication, which has to be considered and controlled.

Through intensive therapy with serum and diuretics, a progressive and complete recovery of kidney function is usually achieved. Rhabdomyolysis is also controlled, observing a decrease in its markers during admission to the Intensive Care Unit.

Before the patient is discharged from hospital, it is advisable to request the Rehabilitation Service to improve leg recovery and normal mobility.

8. Prognosis

The damage is thought to be reversible if the ischemic time is less than 2 hours. When cell death occurs it results in permanent disability (in this order: sensitive nerves, motor nerves, muscle and bone). [17]

Prognosis depends on various factors: injury severity, duration of ischaemia, pre-injury status and comorbidities and, most importantly, time to fasciotomy. [32]

A delay in decompression may lead to 20% of the patients requiring amputation. Muscle necrosis and nerve ischemia lead to permanent neuromuscular dysfunction after the first 12 hours. [16] Other possible sequela is a Volkmann contracture. Exposure of the necrotic muscle after a delayed surgery is associated with loss of the extremity. [17]

In case the diagnosis has been missed or delayed, definitive reconstructive surgery should be postponed. Meanwhile, the patient should be treated through supportive renal therapy until the morbidity has been removed. [32]

From the four compartments of the legs, the loss of one or two can be tolerated. If the patient attends aggressive physical therapy, and also uses ankle-foot braces or splints, he or she can return to normal ambulation eventually. However, if more than two compartments are affected, amputation is sometimes required. The following sequelae are the consequence of nerve injuries: claw or hammer toes, cavus foot, quinovarus, ankle equines, foot drop. All this causes difficulties in the use of footwear, pressure zones as a result of the deformity and impairment of gait. [21]

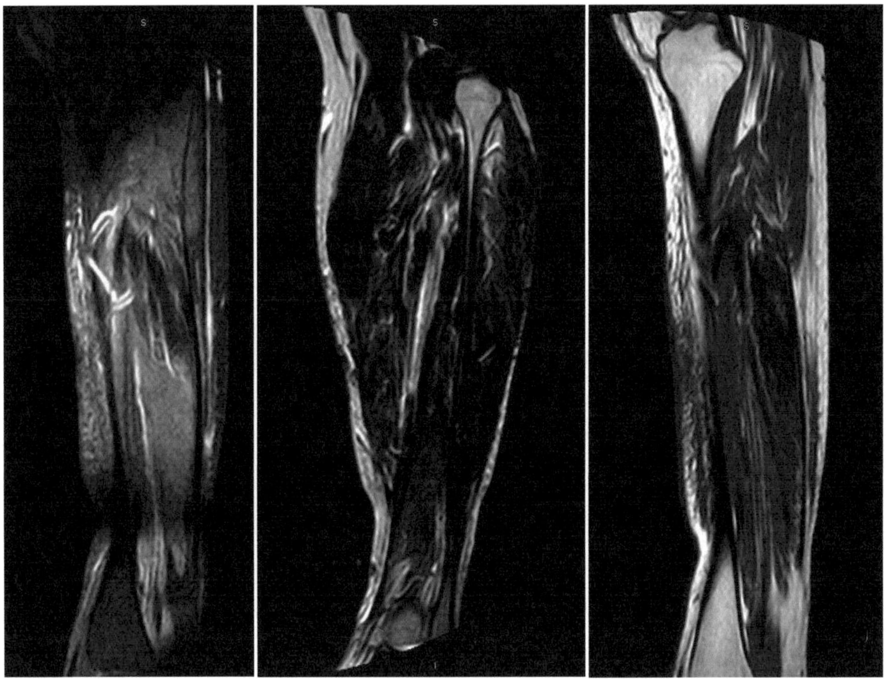

Figure 4.
Magnetic resonance imaging showing sequelae of the compartment syndrome after 6 months: the presence of a certain degree of discrete muscular oedema in a trajectory of approximately 18 cm is observed, affecting the soleus muscles, with a chronic appearance. There is a certain degree of fat infiltration mainly in the proximal third of the muscle mass. Likewise, an apparent degree of scarring and / or fibrosis is also detected in the muscle. The fascia signal is preserved.

Complication	Percentage
Dry scaly skin	40%
Discolored wounds	30%
Tethered scars	26%
Muscle herniation	13%
Pruritus	33%
Swollen limbs	25%
Recurrent ulceration	13%
Tethered tendons	7%
Appearance of scars causing discomfort	23%
Chronic venous insufficiency	—

Table 3.
Fasciotomy complications.

Although the majority of positioning injuries resolve in one month, they may persist beyond 6 months, and the patient may still be needing rehabilitation care. [31] Patient's MRI (Magnetic Resonance Imaging) still shows signs of damage 6 months after the surgery, even in the case of being attending rehabilitation care (**Figure 4**).

In the long-term, reported complication rates of early and late fasciotomies are 4.5% and 54%, respectively (**Table 3**). Pain and altered sensation around the fasciotomy wound occur in 10% and 77%, respectively. [18]

Fasciotomy wounds can cause dry scaly skin in 40% of cases, discolored wounds in 30%, tethered scars in 26%, muscle herniation in 13%, pruritus in 33%, swollen limbs in 25%, recurrent ulceration in 13% and tethered tendons in 7%. Chronic venous insufficiency due to impaired calf muscle pumps may also occur. [21, 32] Appearance of the scars affects 23% of the patients. [17]

Well-leg compartment syndrome may lead to permanent disability and, therefore, has considerable medico-legal implications. This may apply to other rare and life-threatening syndromes during percutaneous nephrolithotomy, such as acute abdominal syndrome. [33]

9. Prevention

Strategies have been developed to prevent the occurrence of this complication, including limitation of the patients' position, optimal medical management of comorbidities before surgery, or even the use of checklists. [18]

In terms of positional preventive measures, the most important thing is to reserve the positioning in extreme Trendelenburg, lithotomy, Trendelenburg or supine Valdivia modified by Galdakao only for when it is necessary. [34] Wrapping of raised legs should be avoided. Intermittent compression is still controversial. It increases the risk of compartment syndrome of the leg, but significantly reduces the occurrence of deep vein thrombosis. Complete passive plantar flexion should be avoided. [17] The use of stirrups has theoretical disadvantages over the use of a split leg table. [18] Positioning the patient's calves just below the level of the right atrium may be beneficial, as it minimizes the degree of elevation of the ankle. [21, 30] It has been advised to remove leg from support every 2 hours for short periods if operating for more than 4 hours. [21]

Overweight patients should be advised to lose weight before the procedure. Other diseases, such as peripheral vascular disease or diabetes, must be optimized. [35] Use of checklists has been shown to help avoid complications by directing attention to risk factors associated with the operation. [18]

Regarding anesthetic issues, we must perform an epidural block with intensity appropriate to the potential pain of the patient. During surgery, the patient must be adequately hydrated, and we must maintain blood pressure in the standard range. [17]

Intraoperative measurement of serum creatine phosphokinase in patients with risk factors who undergo prolonged surgery during ventilation and sedation may be helpful in anticipating an early diagnosis of compartment syndrome of the leg. [21]

In addition, in these types of patients, intraoperative monitoring of compartment pressure could be an option. This monitoring can detect signs of compartment syndrome before the onset of clinical ones. Thus, it could reduce the treatment time for compartment syndrome (fasciotomy) and, therefore, the risk of subsequent complications. [32] If the patient exhibits small elevations, mannitol can be used to induce osmotic diuresis. Additionally, mannitol is as a free radical scavenger. In high risk patients or in prolonged surgeries, urinary pH monitoring allows us to avoid the precipitation of myoglobin and urates, through the infusion of acetazolamide or sodium bicarbonate. [17]

10. Conclusions

Well-leg compartment syndrome is a rare, but potentially devastating complication that may occur during urological surgeries performed in the lithotomy position. It is also possible the development of a compartment syndrome during a percutaneous nephrolithotomy in the Galdakao-modified Supine Valdivia Position.

The factors associated with the development of this complication include: obesity, advanced age, hypertension, hyperlipidemia, diabetes mellitus, combined general-spinal anesthesia, prolonged surgery time and systemic hypotension.

In prolonged surgeries and in patients with risk factors, high levels of awareness of the possibility of this condition are advisable, leading possibly to early treatment. Definitive diagnosis is assessed by directly measuring compartmental pressure.

Early diagnosis and treatment by four compartment fasciotomy is the only way to prevent irreversible damage. Preventive measures reduce the incidence of this condition, which may lead to skin necrosis, permanent neuromuscular dysfunction, myoglobinuric renal failure, amputation and even death.

Conflict of interest

The authors declare no conflict of interest.

Author details

Inés Laso-García*, Fernando Arias-Fúnez, Gemma Duque-Ruiz, David Díaz-Pérez, Alberto Artiles-Medina and Javier Burgos-Revilla
Ramón y Cajal University Hospital, Alcalá University, IRYCIS, Madrid, Spain

*Address all correspondence to: ines.laso.garcia@gmail.com

References

[1] Ljunghall S. Incidence of upper urinary tract stones. Miner Electrolyte Metab [Internet]. 1987 Jan [cited 2015 Jun 1];13(4):220-7. Available from: http://www.ncbi.nlm.nih.gov/pubmed/3306313

[2] Johnson CM, Wilson DM, O'Fallon WM, Malek RS, Kurland LT. Renal stone epidemiology: a 25-year study in Rochester, Minnesota. Kidney Int [Internet]. 1979 Nov [cited 2016 Oct 25];16(5):624-31. Available from: http://www.ncbi.nlm.nih.gov/pubmed/548606

[3] Boyce WH, Garvey FK, Strawcutter HE. Incidence of urinary calculi among patients in general hospitals, 1948 to 1952. J Am Med Assoc [Internet]. 1956 Aug 11 [cited 2016 Oct 25];161(15):1437-42. Available from: http://www.ncbi.nlm.nih.gov/pubmed/13345602

[4] Scales CD, Smith AC, Hanley JM, Saigal CS, Urologic Diseases in America Project. Prevalence of Kidney Stones in the United States. Eur Urol [Internet]. 2012 Jul [cited 2017 Feb 25];62(1):160-5. Available from: http://www.ncbi.nlm.nih.gov/pubmed/22498635

[5] Ramello A, Vitale C, Marangella M. Epidemiology of nephrolithiasis. J Nephrol [Internet]. 2000 [cited 2017 Mar 27];13 Suppl 3:S45-50. Available from: http://www.ncbi.nlm.nih.gov/pubmed/11132032

[6] Decoster M, Bigot JC, Carre JL, Morin JF, Mahé JL, Tanquerel T, et al. [Epidemiologic study of urinary calculi in Western France]. Presse Med [Internet]. 2002 Jan 26 [cited 2016 Oct 25];31(3):113-8. Available from: http://www.ncbi.nlm.nih.gov/pubmed/11859735

[7] Turney BW, Reynard JM, Noble JG, Keoghane SR. Trends in urological stone disease. BJU Int [Internet]. 2012 Apr [cited 2017 Feb 13];109(7):1082-7. Available from: http://www.ncbi.nlm.nih.gov/pubmed/21883851

[8] Zhao F, Li J, Tang L, Li C. A comparative study of endoscopic combined intrarenal surgery (ECIRS) in the galdakao-modified supine valdivia (GMSV) position and minimally invasive percutaneous nephrolithotomy for complex nephrolithiasis: a retrospective single-center study. Urolithiasis [Internet]. Springer; 2020 [cited 2021 Feb 1];Aug 10. Available from: https://pubmed.ncbi.nlm.nih.gov/32776245/

[9] Melo PA de S, Vicentini FC, Perrella R, Murta CB, Claro JF de A. Comparative study of percutaneous nephrolithotomy performed in the traditional prone position and in three different supine positions. Int Braz J Urol [Internet]. Brazilian Society of Urology; 2019 Jan 1 [cited 2021 Feb 1];45(1):108-17. Available from: https://pubmed.ncbi.nlm.nih.gov/30521168/

[10] Scoffone CM, Cracco CM. Invited review: the tale of ECIRS (Endoscopic Combined IntraRenal Surgery) in the Galdakao-modified supine Valdivia position [Internet]. Urolithiasis. Springer Verlag; 2018 [cited 2021 Jan 31]. p. 115-23. Available from: https://pubmed.ncbi.nlm.nih.gov/29189885/

[11] Ibarluzea G, Scoffone CM, Cracco CM, Poggio M, Porpiglia F, Terrone C, et al. Supine Valdivia and modified lithotomy position for simultaneous anterograde and retrograde endourological access. BJU Int [Internet]. 2007 Jul [cited 2019 Oct 15];100(1):233-6. Available from: http://doi.wiley.com/10.1111/j.1464-410X.2007.06960.x

[12] Cohen SA, Hurt WG. Compartment syndrome associated with lithotomy

position and intermittent compression stockings. Obstet Gynecol. 2001;97(5):832-3.

[13] Clarke D, Mullings S, Franklin S, Jones K. Well leg compartment syndrome. Trauma Case Reports. Elsevier Ltd; 2017 Oct 1;11:5-7.

[14] Pfeffer SD, Halliwill JR, Warner MA. Effects of lithotomy position and external compression on lower leg muscle compartment pressure. Anesthesiology [Internet]. 2001 Sep [cited 2019 Oct 15];95(3):632-6. Available from: https://insights.ovid.com/crossref?an=00000542-200109000-00014

[15] Gill M, Fligelstone L, Keating J, Jayne DG, Renton S, Shearman CP, et al. Avoiding, diagnosing and treating well leg compartment syndrome after pelvic surgery. Br J Surg. John Wiley and Sons Ltd; 2019 Aug 1;106(9):1156-66.

[16] Mattei A, Di Pierro GB, Rafeld V, Konrad C, Beutler J, Danuser H. Positioning Injury, Rhabdomyolysis, and Serum Creatine Kinase-Concentration Course in Patients Undergoing Robot-Assisted Radical Prostatectomy and Extended Pelvic Lymph Node Dissection. J Endourol [Internet]. 2013 Jan [cited 2019 Oct 15];27(1):45-51. Available from: http://www.liebertpub.com/doi/10.1089/end.2012.0169

[17] Mabvuure NT, Malahias M, Hindocha S, Khan W, Juma A. Acute Compartment Syndrome of the Limbs: Current Concepts and Management. Open Orthop J [Internet]. 2012 Nov 30 [cited 2019 Oct 15];6(1):535-43. Available from: https://openorthopaedicsjournal.com/VOLUME/6/PAGE/535/

[18] Mumtaz FH, Chew H, Gelister JS. Lower limb compartment syndrome associated with the lithotomy position: Concepts and perspectives for the urologist. BJU Int. 2002;90(8):792-9.

[19] Sukhu T, Krupski TL. Patient positioning and prevention of injuries in patients undergoing laparoscopic and robot-assisted urologic procedures. Curr Urol Rep [Internet]. 2014 Apr 27 [cited 2019 Oct 15];15(4):398. Available from: http://link.springer.com/10.1007/s11934-014-0398-1

[20] Chung JH, Ahn KR, Park JH, Kim CS, Kang KS, Yoo SH, et al. Lower leg compartment syndrome following prolonged orthopedic surgery in the lithotomy position -A case report-. Korean J Anesthesiol [Internet]. 2010 Dec [cited 2020 Apr 21];59 Suppl(SUPPL.):S49-52. Available from: http://www.ncbi.nlm.nih.gov/pubmed/21286459

[21] RAZA A, BYRNE D, TOWNELL N. Lower Limb (Well Leg) Compartment Syndrome After Urological Pelvic Surgery. J Urol [Internet]. 2004 Jan [cited 2019 Oct 15];171(1):5-11. Available from: http://www.ncbi.nlm.nih.gov/pubmed/14665832

[22] Simms MS, Terry TR. Well leg compartment syndrome after pelvic and perineal surgery in the lithotomy position. Postgraduate Medical Journal. 2005. p. 534-6.

[23] Wassenaar EB, van den Brand JGH, van der Werken C. Compartment syndrome of the lower leg after surgery in the modified lithotomy position: report of seven cases. Dis *Colon rectum* [Internet]. 2006 Sep [cited 2019 Oct 15];49(9):1449-53. Available from: https://insights.ovid.com/crossref?an=00003453-200649090-00025

[24] Chin KY, Hemington-Gorse SJ, Darcy CM. Bilateral well leg compartment syndrome associated with lithotomy (Lloyd Davies) position during gastrointestinal surgery: a case report and review of literature. Eplasty [Internet]. 2009 Oct 14 [cited 2020 Apr 21];9:e48. Available from: http://www.ncbi.nlm.nih.gov/pubmed/19915657

[25] Yamamoto T, Fujie A, Tanikawa H, Funayama A, Fukuda K. Bilateral Well Leg Compartment Syndrome Localized in the Anterior and Lateral Compartments following Urologic Surgery in Lithotomy Position. Case Rep Orthop [Internet]. 2018 Nov 14 [cited 2019 Oct 15];2018:1-4. Available from: http://www.ncbi.nlm.nih.gov/pubmed/30538877

[26] Tison C, Périgaud C, Vrignaud S, Capelli M, Lehur PA. Syndrome bilatéral des loges de jambe après chirurgie colorectale en position à double équipe. Ann Chir. 2002 Sep;127(7):535-8.

[27] Rosevear HM, Lightfoot AJ, Zahs M, Waxman SW, Winfield HN. Lessons learned from a case of calf compartment syndrome after robot-assisted laparoscopic prostatectomy. J Endourol [Internet]. 2010 Oct [cited 2019 Oct 15];24(10):1597-601. Available from: http://www.liebertpub.com/doi/10.1089/end.2009.0666

[28] Wollin DA, Preminger GM. Percutaneous nephrolithotomy: complications and how to deal with them. Urolithiasis. Springer Verlag; 2018. p. 87-97.

[29] Tao J, Sheng L, Zhang H jie, Chen R, Sun Z quan, Qian W qing. Acute Abdominal Compartment Syndrome as a Complication of Percutaneous Nephrolithotomy: Two Cases Reports and Literature Review. Urol Case Reports. Elsevier Inc; 2016 Sep 1;8:12-4.

[30] Mizuno J, Takahashi T. Male sex, height, weight, and body mass index can increase external pressure to calf region using knee-crutch-type leg holder system in lithotomy position. Ther Clin Risk Manag [Internet]. 2016 Feb [cited 2019 Oct 15];12:305. Available from: http://www.ncbi.nlm.nih.gov/pubmed/26955278

[31] Romero FR, Pilati R, Kulysz D, Canali FA V, Baggio P V, Brenny Filho T. [Combined risk factors leading to well-leg compartment syndrome after laparoscopic radical prostatectomy]. Actas Urol Esp [Internet]. 2009 Sep [cited 2019 Oct 15];33(8):920-4. Available from: http://www.ncbi.nlm.nih.gov/pubmed/19900389

[32] Mills JT, Burris MB, Warburton DJ, Conaway MR, Schenkman NS, Krupski TL. Positioning injuries associated with robotic assisted urological surgery. J Urol. 2013 Aug;190(2):580-4.

[33] Donaldson J, Haddad B, Khan WS. The Pathophysiology, Diagnosis and Current Management of Acute Compartment Syndrome. Open Orthop J. Bentham Science Publishers Ltd.; 2014 Jul 17;8(1):185-93.

[34] Googe B, Lackey AE, Arnold PA, Vick LR. The Modified Lithotomy: A Surgical Position for Lower Extremity Wound Care Procedures in Super Morbidly Obese Patients. A Case Study. Wound Manag Prev [Internet]. 2019 Jul [cited 2020 Apr 21];65(7):30-4. Available from: http://www.ncbi.nlm.nih.gov/pubmed/31373561

[35] Takechi K, Kitamura S, Shimizu I, Yorozuya T. Lower limb perfusion during robotic-assisted laparoscopic radical prostatectomy evaluated by near-infrared spectroscopy: an observational prospective study. BMC Anesthesiol [Internet]. BioMed Central Ltd.; 2018 Aug 18 [cited 2020 Apr 21];18(1):114. Available from: http://www.ncbi.nlm.nih.gov/pubmed/30121089